Physical Signs in Orthopedic and Neurologic Disorders

Roger Pillemer

Physical Signs in Orthopedic and Neurologic Disorders

A Practical Guide

Springer

Roger Pillemer
Cammeray, NSW, Australia

ISBN 978-3-031-99528-6 ISBN 978-3-031-99529-3 (eBook)
https://doi.org/10.1007/978-3-031-99529-3

This Springer imprint is published by the registered company Springer Nature Switzerland AG
The registered company address is: Gewerbestrasse 11, 6330 Cham, Switzerland

To our grandchildren, Ben, Max, Noah, Lucas, Mya, Lachlan, Cole, Grayson, and Lilah Jayne Pillemer, and Mia and Theo Weigler, and to their parents who have all brought us so much pride and joy.

Preface

> *Live as if you were to die tomorrow. Learn as if you were to live forever.* –Mahatma Gandhi

Among the most exciting things in my life has been learning new things. Either by instruction or reading, but particularly from experience.

After almost 60 years in clinical practice, the last 15 or so in medicolegal work, I am as excited today as I have ever been, to learn something new.

And this applies particularly to finding and appreciating physical signs, which many would still view as the basis of medicine. Unfortunately, with the advent of highly sophisticated methods of investigation, now including AI, this skill is being progressively lost.

The other aspect of physical signs that I would like to stress is the importance of the following: 'If you do not think of it, you will not look for it. And if you do not look for it, you will never find it.'

So, this book is a collection of signs, ideas and concepts which have all given me 'aha' moments in the past. It is the sort of book that I would love to have read!

I hope that you will find items of interest and excitement in these unrelated chapters, all of which are based on examination and clinical findings.

I have included an additional chapter on 'Tips and Time-Savers in Medicolegal Reporting'.

And I hope that you will enjoy reading the book as much as I have enjoyed writing it!

Cammeray, NSW, Australia
January 2025

Roger Pillemer

Acknowledgements A special thank you to Dr Brian Noll, Orthopaedic Surgeon, colleague and friend, for his advice and support for every one of my endeavours over the past 20 years, including his significant contribution to this book.

To Dr Jerry Jersky, friend and mentor, for encouragement and guidance since my first days as an intern and until the present.

Thank you to Dr Andreas Loefler, Dr Hari Kapilla, Dr Doron Sher, Dr Todd Gothelf and Dr David Crocker for reading over their special interest areas in the book and making many helpful suggestions. All errors are my own.

And to Ruth Hadfield for her enormous help and advice in the preparation of this book.

And special thanks to my wife Margie for her love, friendship and tolerance for over 50 years.

Contents

About the Author

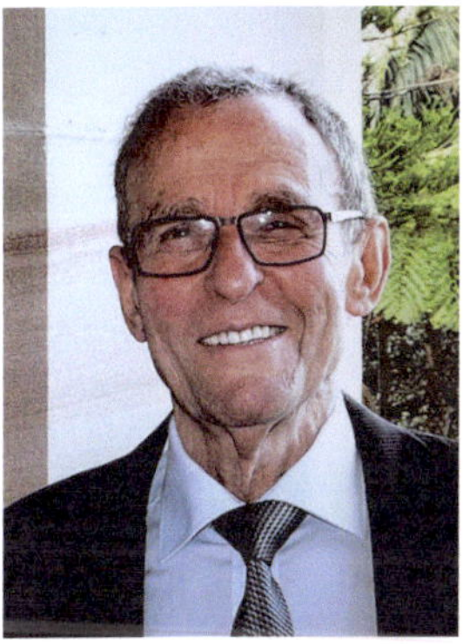

Roger Pillemer, OAM, MBBCh, FRCS, FRACS, FAOrthA is an orthopaedic surgeon who did his early training in South Africa and the UK. He was a 1974 ABC Travelling Fellow who is now resident in Australia. He has always had a passion for teaching.

His previous books in the series are:

Handbook of Upper Extremity Examination, Springer 2022 and

Handbook of Lumbar Spine and Lower Extremity Examination, Springer 2023.

Roger also has a YouTube series on the importance of physical signs.

1 The Median Nerve

This chapter will be discussed under the following headings:

A. Anatomy
B. Function
C. Testing for median nerve function
   (a) Motor
   (b) Sensory
D. Lesions of the median nerve
E. Differentiation between high and low median nerve lesions

1.1 Anatomy

- The median nerve arises from the medial and lateral cords of the brachial plexus; it is one of the five terminal branches of the plexus* (Fig. 1.1).
- It contains fibres from C5 to T1.
- In the upper arm, the nerve lies lateral to the brachial artery, then crosses in front of the artery to lie on its medial side at the elbow, both structures being medial to the biceps tendon in the cubital fossa (Fig. 1.2).
- In the forearm, the nerve passes between the two heads of pronator teres, and beneath the fibrous arch of flexor digitorum superficialis (FDS) to lie on flexor digitorum profundus (FDP) (Fig. 1.3).

R. Pillemer, *Physical Signs in Orthopedic and Neurologic Disorders*, https://doi.org/10.1007/978-3-031-99529-3_1

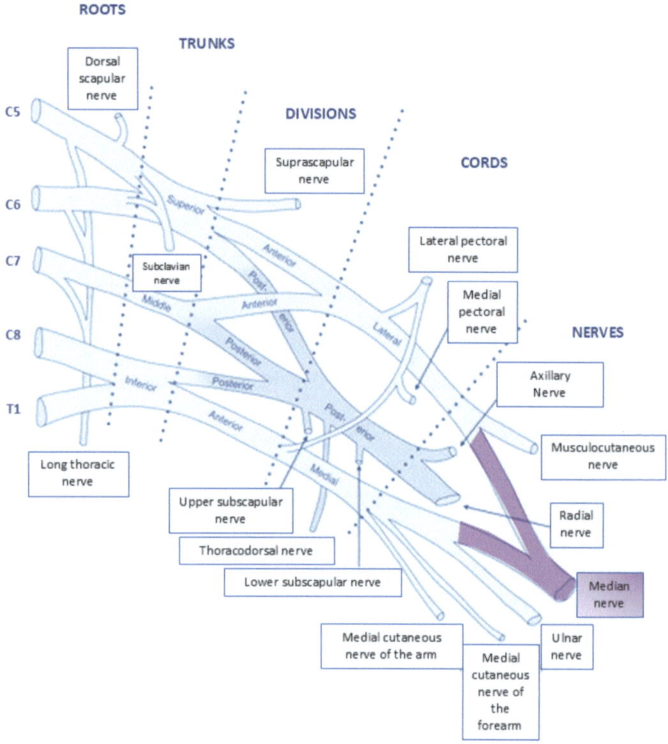

Fig. 1.1 Median nerve

- The anterior interosseous nerve arises in the proximal forearm and runs along the volar surface of FDP terminating in the volar wrist joint capsule where it gives sensory fibres.
- Closer to the wrist, the median nerve becomes more superficial, running behind and lateral to the tendon of palmaris longus.
- It then passes beneath the transverse carpal ligament to enter the palm of the hand where it divides into motor and sensory branches (Fig. 1.4).

*The other four terminal branches being the musculocutaneous, ulnar, axillary, and radial nerves.

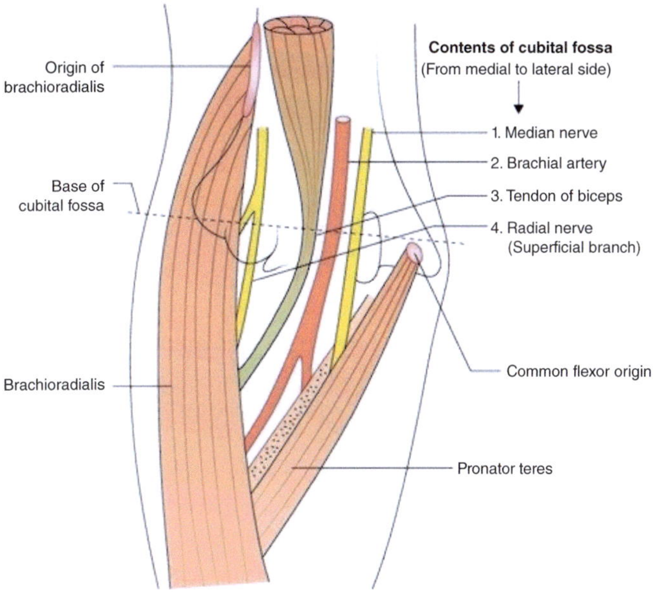

Fig. 1.2 Right arm: median nerve medial to the brachial artery

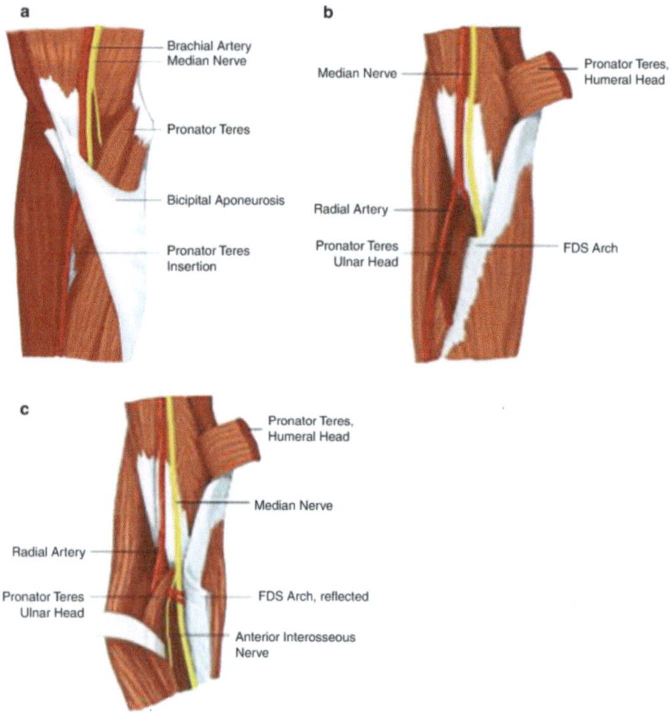

Fig. 1.3 Median nerve passing between the two heads of pronator teres and beneath the fibrous arch of FDS: (**a**) Pronator Teres: two heads. (**b**) FDS arch. (**c**) FDS arch reflected: anterior interosseous nerve (AIN)

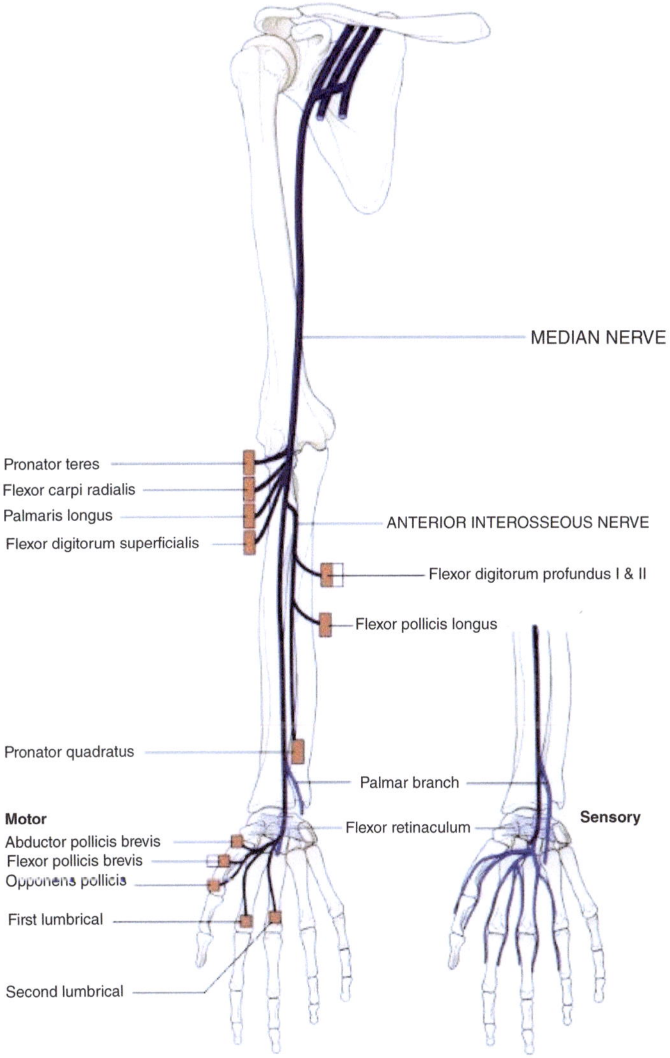

Fig. 1.4 Motor and sensory branches of the median nerve

1.2 Function

1.2.1 Motor

- Figure 1.4
- The median nerve supplies all the flexor muscles in the forearm, except for flexor carpi ulnaris and the ulnar head of FDP (and therefore innervates the radial head of FDP, flexor pollicis longus (FPL), FDS, flexor carpi radialis, pronator teres, and palmaris longus).
- The anterior interosseous nerve (AIN) is a branch of the median nerve, which supplies the radial head of FDP and flexor pollicis longus (FPL).

The motor branches in the hand supply the muscles of the thenar eminence and the lateral two lumbricals.**

**Mnemonic for the intrinsic muscles supplies by the median nerve: 'LOAF':

- *L*ateral two lumbricals
- *O*pponens pollicis
- *A*bductor pollicis brevis
- *F*lexor pollicis brevis

1.2.2 Sensory

- Sensory branches supply the skin of the palm and the palmar surface of the lateral 3½ digits, as well as the distal part of the dorsal aspect of these digits as far as the middle phalanges (Fig. 1.5).
- Note that the palmar cutaneous branch arises in the distal forearm passing superficial to the flexor retinaculum, to supply the skin of the proximal palm and thenar eminence (Fig. 1.6).***

***Important in differentiating high and low median nerve lesions (see below).

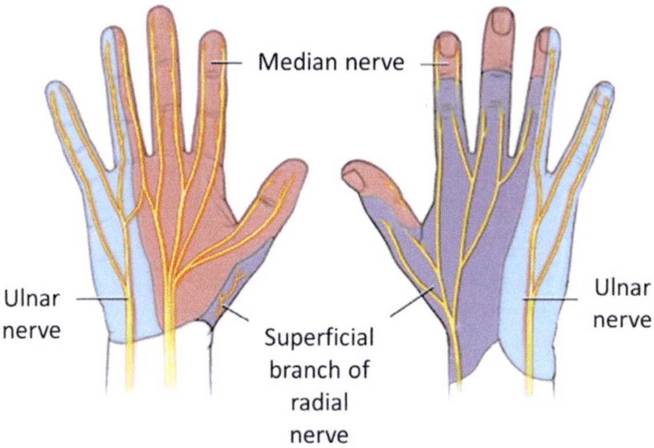

Fig. 1.5 Sensory innervation of the hand

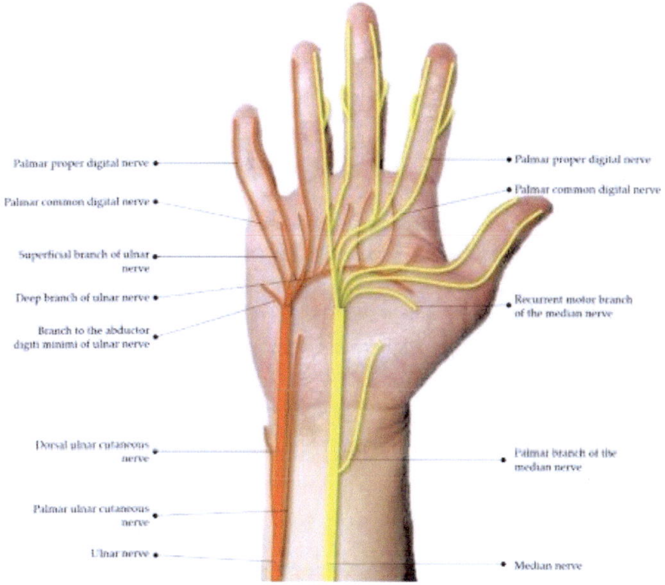

Fig. 1.6 Palmar cutaneous branch

1.3 Testing for Median Nerve Motor Function

1.3.1 Extrinsic

- Flexor digitorum profundus attaches to the base of the distal phalanx of each finger; it is the only tendon that flexes the DIP joint.
- To isolate the profundus action, hold the MP and PIP joints in extension, thereby overcoming any superficialis action.
- Any flexion that now occurs at the DIP joint is therefore due to profundus action only (Fig. 1.7).
- Test all four fingers and the thumb (flexor pollicis longus) in this way (Fig. 1.8).
- The method of isolating the superficialis function is to hold three of the four fingers in full extension, thereby preventing any profundus action.

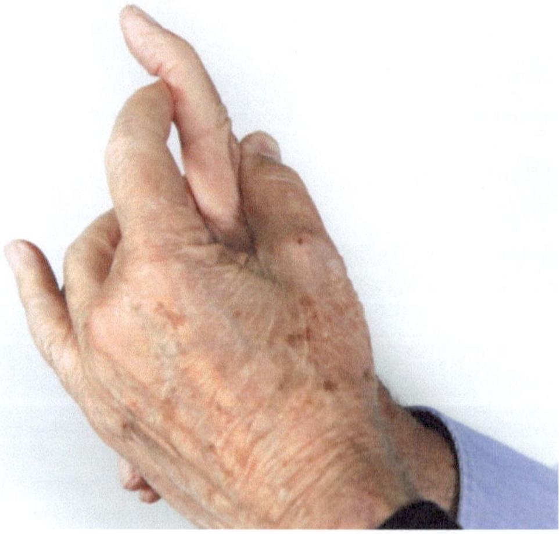

Fig. 1.7 Isolation of profundus action

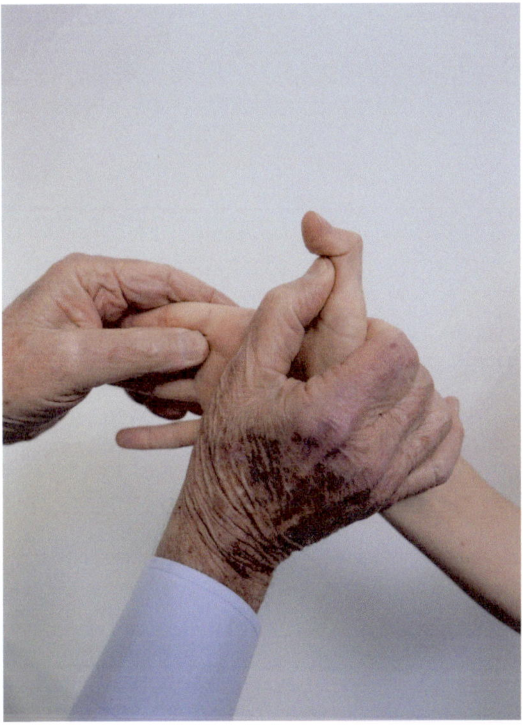

Fig. 1.8 Testing flexor pollicis longus

- Flexing the finger now occurs at the level of the PIP joint and is due to the action of superficialis only (Fig. 1.9). Test this on yourself and note how the DIP joint is 'floppy'.
- Test each finger in this way.

1.3.2 Intrinsic

- There are three 'tests' for median nerve intrinsic motor function:
  - Abduction of the thumb—ask the patient to place the hand in supination and lift the thumb towards the roof, against resistance (Fig. 1.10). Feel the contraction.

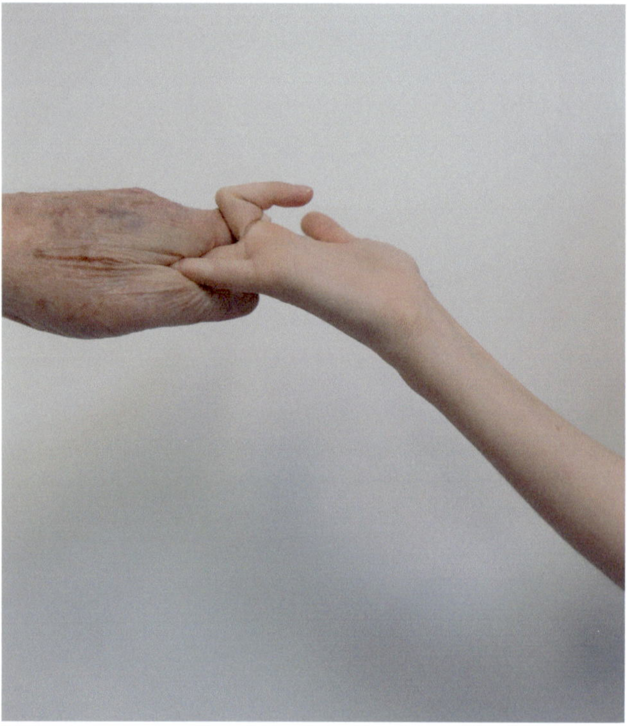

Fig. 1.9 Isolating the superficialis function

- Opposition of the thumb—ask the patient to pinch the tip of the thumb and index finger together. Try to overcome this (Fig. 1.11).
- Wasting of the thenar eminence—always check for this (Fig. 1.12).

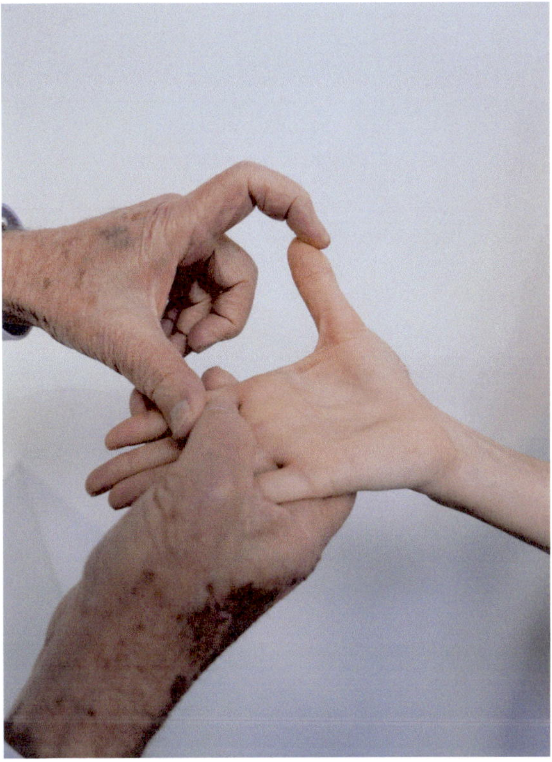

Fig. 1.10 Abduction of the thumb

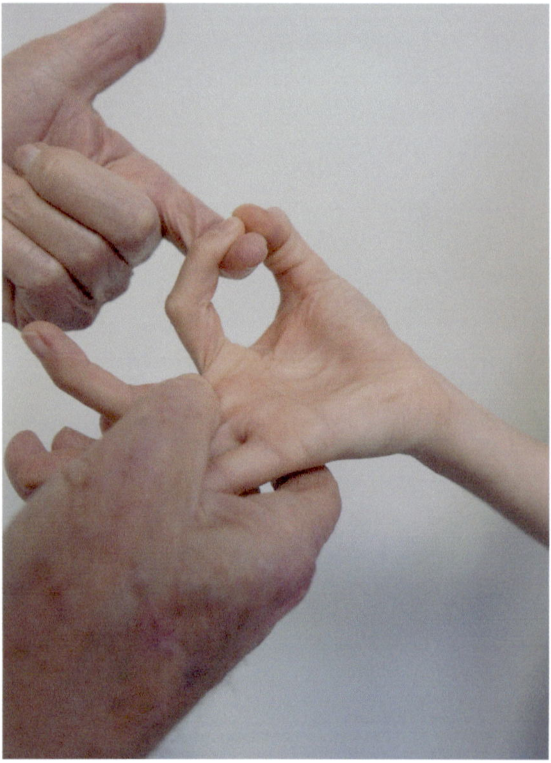

Fig. 1.11 Opposition of the thumb

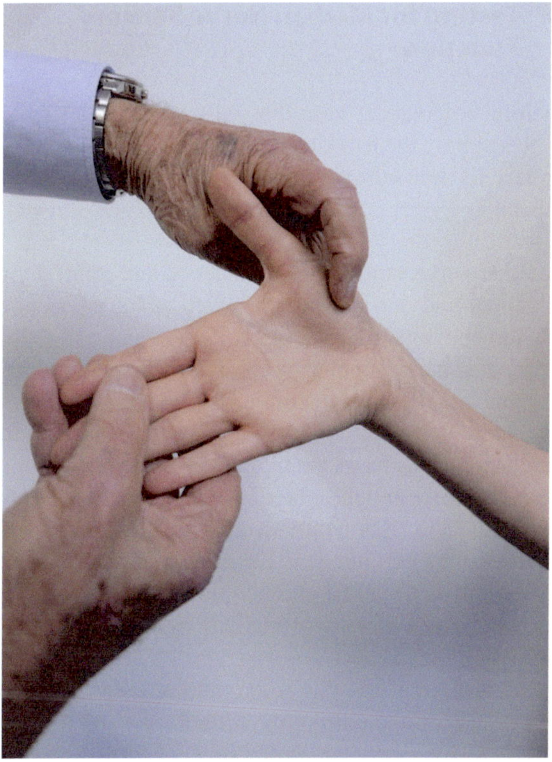

Fig. 1.12 Thenar eminence

1.4 Testing for Median Nerve Sensory Function

It is helpful to consider here the sensory function of the three nerves that supply the hand, the radial, ulnar, and median nerves.

Figure 1.13 shows the commonly accepted sensory innervation of the hand.

- The ulnar nerve supplies the medial one and a half digits both the palmar and dorsal aspects, as well as the adjacent part of the palm and dorsum of the hand.
- The median nerve supplies the rest of the palmar aspect of the hand and supplies the dorsum of the distal part of the lateral three and a half digits to a level somewhere between the DIP and PIP joints (as far as the middle phalanges).
- The radial nerve supplies the rest of the dorsum of the hand.
- Despite the description provided above, there is some overlap of the sensory regions. It is therefore important to note that there are also so-called autonomous zones which are those areas very specifically supplied by a particular nerve (Fig. 1.14).
- For the median nerve, this is the pulp of the index finger; for the ulnar nerve, the pulp of the little finger; and for the radial

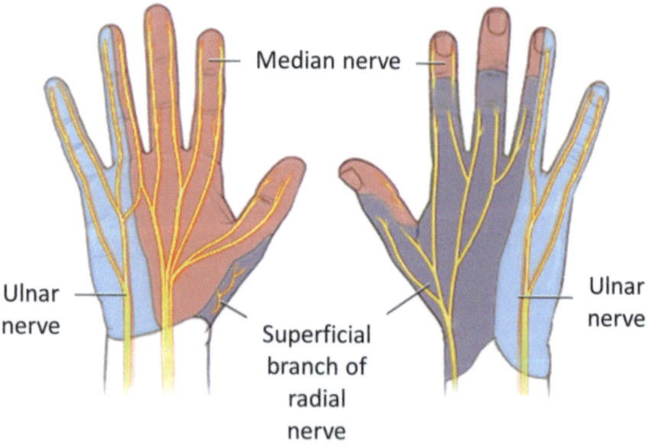

Fig. 1.13 Sensory innervation of the hand

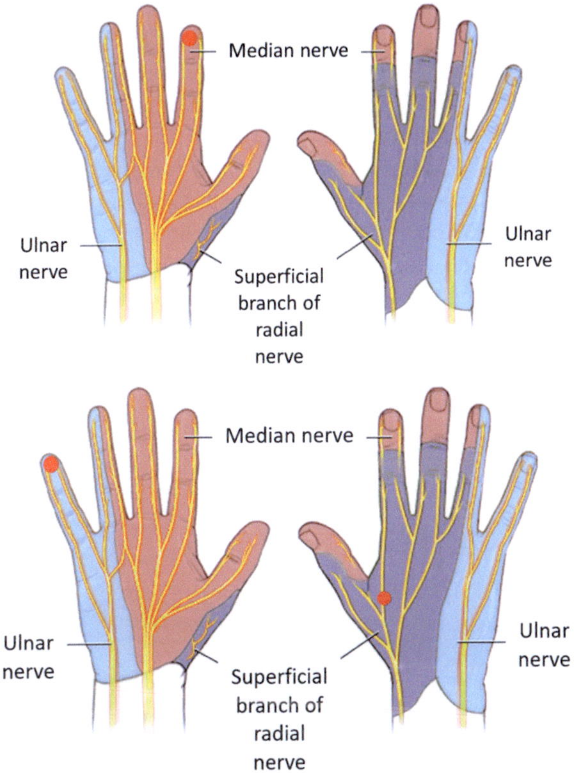

Fig. 1.14 Sensory innervation of the hand

nerve, it is the web space on the dorsum of the hand between the thumb and index finger.

As with sensory testing in general, this needs to be carried out slowly and deliberately. The patient needs to understand what you are doing and needs enough time to consider and respond. Sensory testing needs to be repeated if there is any doubt and always compared to the opposite side.

How is sensation in the hand tested in a patient who is unconscious or a child who is too young to understand? Here are three suggestions:

- With nerve damage, there is loss of autonomic supply to the fingers and loss of sudomotor function (sweating). As a result, the pulp of the affected digit or digits feels dry when compared to the unaffected fingers. Telling the difference requires careful examination and practice!
- The so-called violin test, carried out by running a smooth plastic object such as a pen over the digit, helps to identify loss of sensation. With normal sensation, and therefore, normal sweating, running a smooth object over the digit is associated with a feeling of slight resistance because of the moisture (Fig. 1.15). When sensation is lost and the skin is dry (due to lack of sweat-

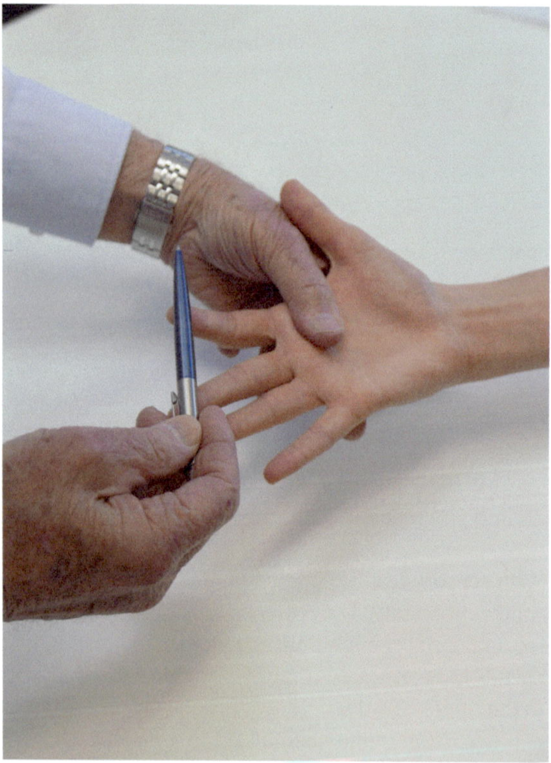

Fig. 1.15 The violin test

ing), there is much less resistance. This can be illustrated by doing the test on one's own normal finger and repeating it after placing a piece of tissue paper between the digit and the pen (Fig. 1.16).

- The 'prune test': If you have spent a lot of time in water, you will have noticed how the skin of the pulp of the fingers tends to wrinkle (Fig. 1.17). This does not happen in denervated digits. The mechanism is thought to be due to vasoconstriction and there is much discussion as to the evolutionary reason for this.

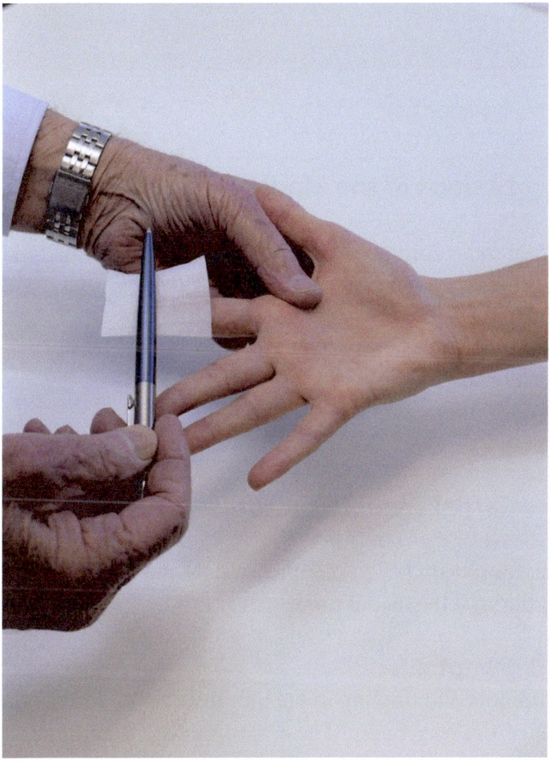

Fig. 1.16 The violin test with tissue paper

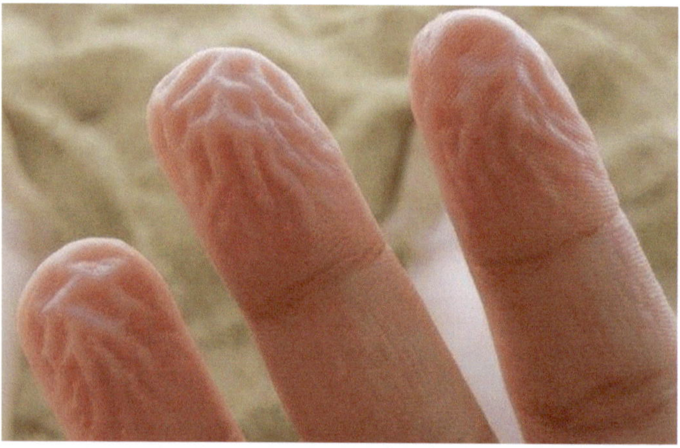

Fig. 1.17 Prune test

1.5 Lesions of the Median Nerve

The three most common and well-known entrapment syndromes are as follows:

- Carpal tunnel syndrome
- Pronator teres syndrome
- Anterior interosseous syndrome

1.5.1 Carpal Tunnel Syndrome

This condition is due to compression of the median nerve as it passes through the carpal tunnel (Fig. 1.18).

1.5.1.1 Symptoms

- Numbness and tingling in the thumb, index, middle, and radial side of the ring finger. These symptoms are particularly troublesome at night and in the early morning.
- Occasionally patients report that they drop things during the day.
- Pain in more severe cases.

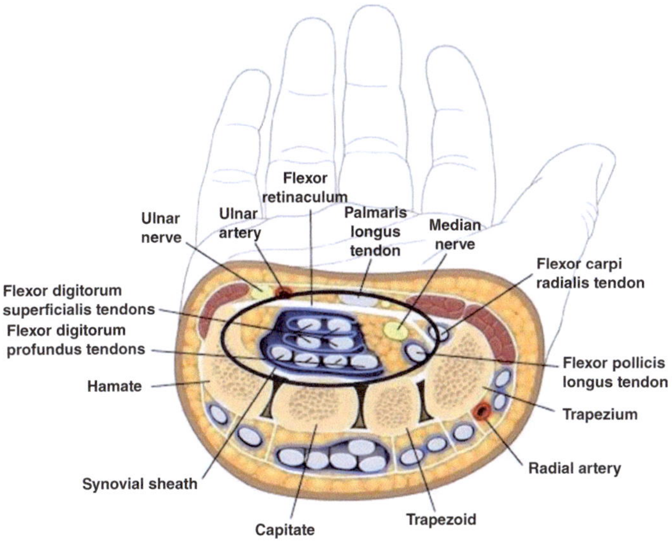

Fig. 1.18 Carpal tunnel

1.5.1.2 Physical Signs

- Tinel's sign: parasthesias reproduced by tapping over the carpal tunnel (Fig. 1.19).
- Phalen's test: parasthesias reproduced by holding the wrists flexed for 30–60 s (Fig. 1.20). In severe cases, symptoms may occur within 10 s or less.
- Durkan's test: symptoms reproduced by direct pressure over the carpal tunnel using the examiner's thumb (Fig. 1.21).
- Weakness or wasting of muscles of the thenar eminence supplied by the median nerve in advanced cases.

1.5.2 Pronator Teres Syndrome

Compression of the median nerve between the two heads of pronator teres muscle.

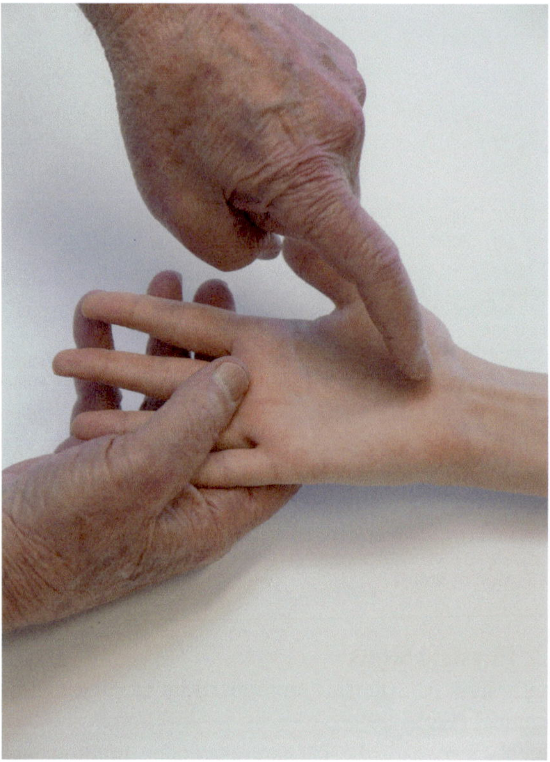

Fig. 1.19 Tinel's sign

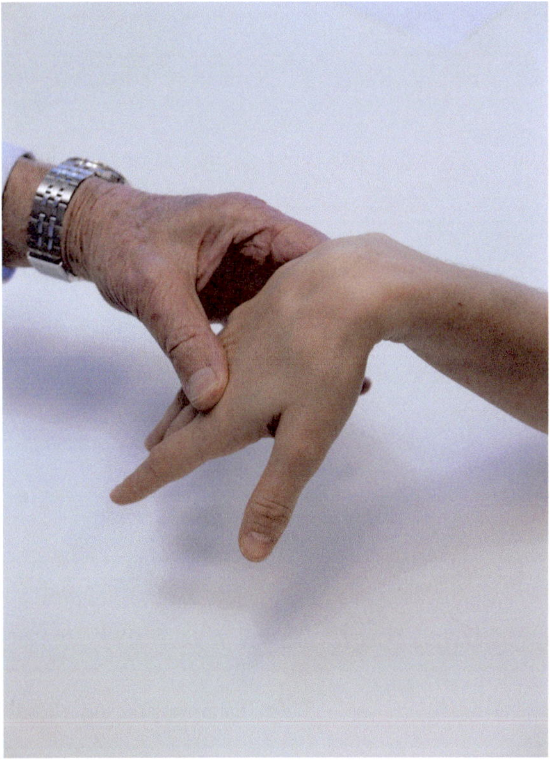

Fig. 1.20 Phalen's test

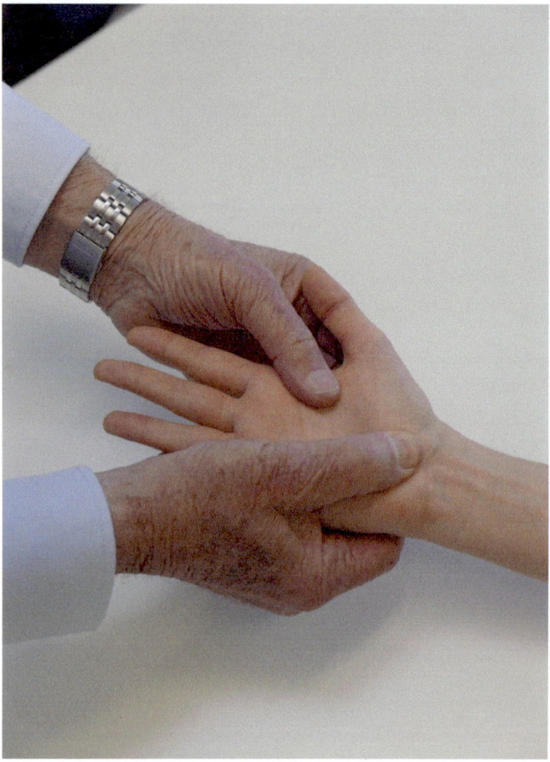

Fig. 1.21 Durkan's test

- Pain in the proximal volar forearm.
- Positive Tinel's sign in proximal volar forearm.
- Sensory changes in the palmar cutaneous branch of the median nerve, as well as parasthesias in the thumb, index, middle, and radial half of the ring finger.

1.5.3 Anterior Interosseous Nerve Syndrome: (AIN)

The AIN is a purely motor branch of the median nerve—the syndrome therefore results in a pure motor neuropathy.

- Causes an isolated palsy of flexor pollicis longus, and FDP to the index and middle fingers, and pronator quadratus.
- May therefore result in the inability to make the 'OK' sign (Fig. 1.22) which involves flexing the IP joint of the thumb and the DIP joint of the index finger.
- Any attempt to 'tip pinch' will result in a 'pulp pinch' (Fig. 1.23).

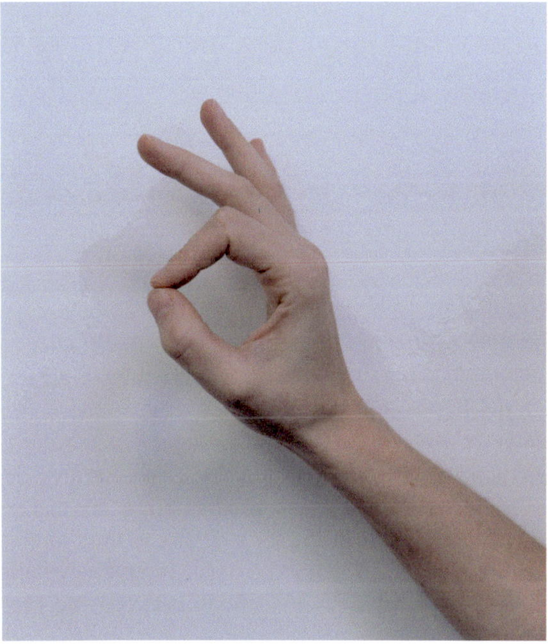

Fig. 1.22 OK sign

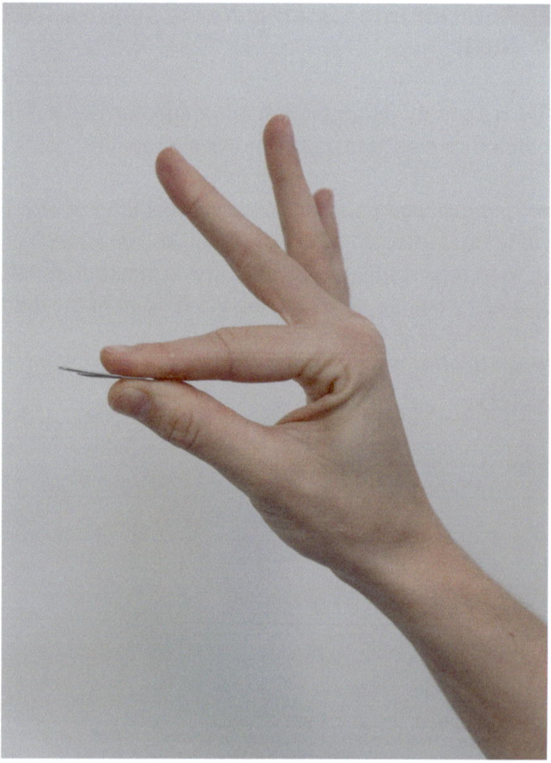

Fig. 1.23 Pulp pinch

1.5.4 Additional Notes

- High median nerve lesions above mid-forearm may result in the 'Benediction sign' when attempting to make a fist (Fig. 1.24) with loss of the long flexors to the thumb, index, and middle fingers. The middle finger is passively pulled into flexion because of the connections between the profundus tendons.
- It is worth noting that an ulnar nerve lesion may result in a similar posture when attempting to extend the fingers.
- While carpal tunnel compression is common, the more proximal compressive lesions are rare.

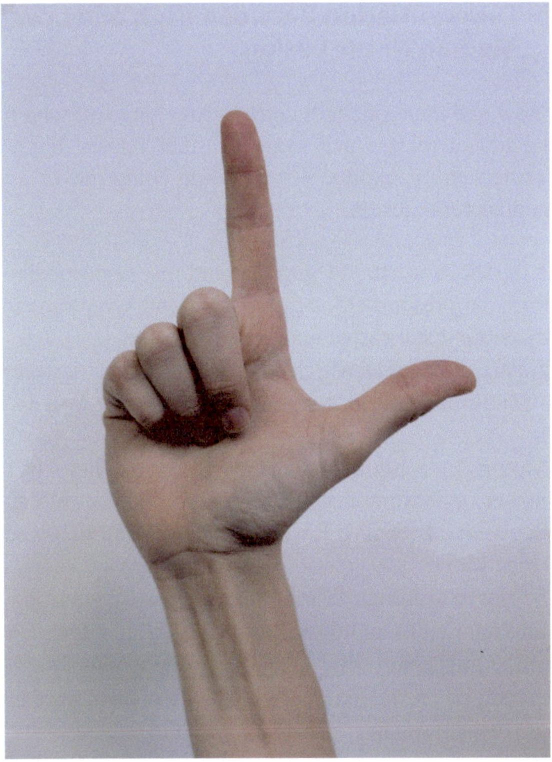

Fig. 1.24 Benediction sign

- Other causes of proximal compression include Struther's ligament, the bicipital aponeurosis (Lacertus tunnel syndrome), and the proximal edge of FDS.
- Injury to the median nerve can occur anywhere between the hand and the brachial plexus.
- Another cause of a low median nerve lesion is damage to the recurrent branch in the hand which causes denervation of flexor pollicis brevis, opponens pollicis, and abductor pollicis brevis, with loss of muscle mass of the thenar eminence; a so-called ape hand. Importantly there is no sensory loss, and this lesion may well be missed if motor function is not tested for specifically.

1.6 Differentiation Between High and Low Median Nerve Lesions

Every now and then, one will come across a patient who has had a carpal tunnel release and even a further release but with no improvement in symptoms, the condition being due to a missed high median nerve lesion.

- It is therefore worth keeping in mind that high median nerve lesions can present with similar signs and symptoms to those of the more distal carpal tunnel compression.
- There are three signs which clearly distinguish between these two conditions, one motor and one sensory, as well as Tinel's sign:
  - Motor: In a high median nerve lesion, there is loss of power of flexion of the IP joint of the thumb (FPL), which does not occur in a low lesion (carpal tunnel syndrome) (Fig. 1.25).
  - Sensory: In a high lesion, there is loss of sensation in the proximal palm and thenar eminence which does not occur in the low lesion (Fig. 1.26), because the palmar cutaneous branch of the median nerve enters the palm superficial to the carpal tunnel.
  - In high lesions, a positive Tinel's sign occurs at a more proximal level.
  - High lesions may also include the 'Benediction sign', and the inability to make the 'OK' sign.

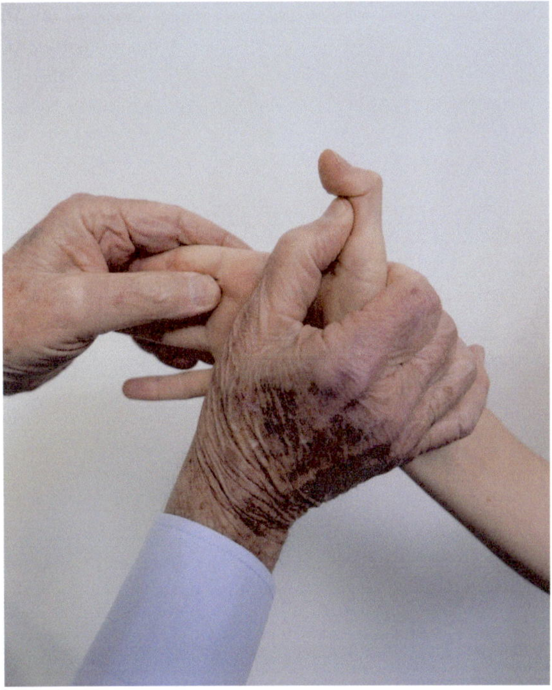

Fig. 1.25 High lesion

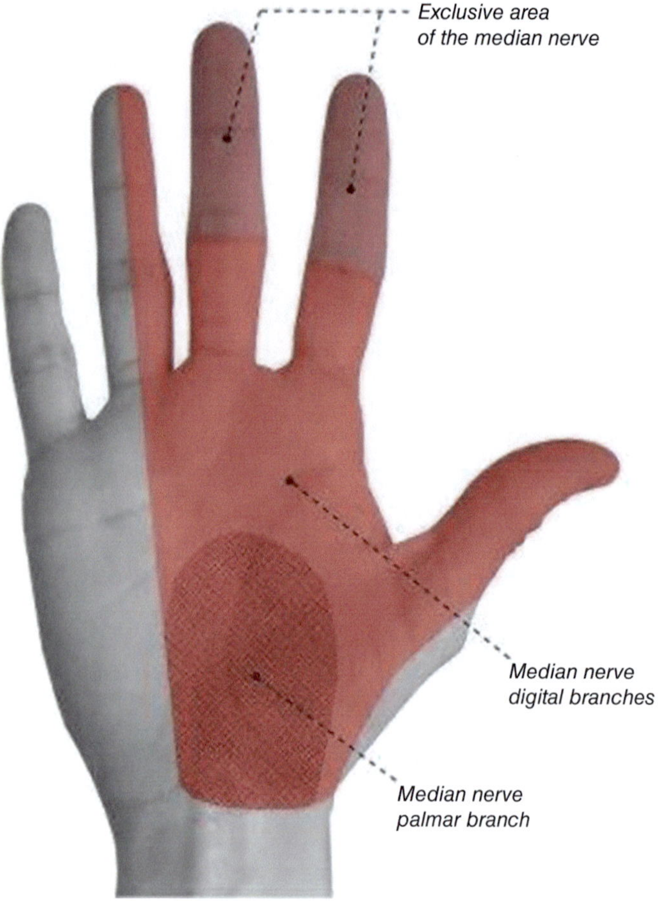

Fig. 1.26 Loss of sensation in high lesion

The Ulnar Nerve 2

This chapter will be discussed under the following headings:

A. Anatomy
B. Function
C. Testing for ulnar nerve function
D. Lesions of the ulnar nerve
E. Explanation of the deformity in the ulnar claw hand
F. The ulnar paradox

2.1 Anatomy

- The ulnar nerve arises from the medial cord of the brachial in the axilla; it is one of the five terminal branches of the plexus* (Fig. 2.1).
- It contains fibres from spinal nerve roots C8 and T1.
- It passes down the medial aspect of the arm lying between the axillary artery and vein, piercing the intermuscular fascia to enter the posterior compartment (Fig. 2.2).
- It then passes behind the medial epicondyle in the ulnar groove and then between the two heads of flexor carpi ulnaris (Fig. 2.3) to enter the flexor compartment of the forearm.

R. Pillemer, *Physical Signs in Orthopedic and Neurologic Disorders*, https://doi.org/10.1007/978-3-031-99529-3_2

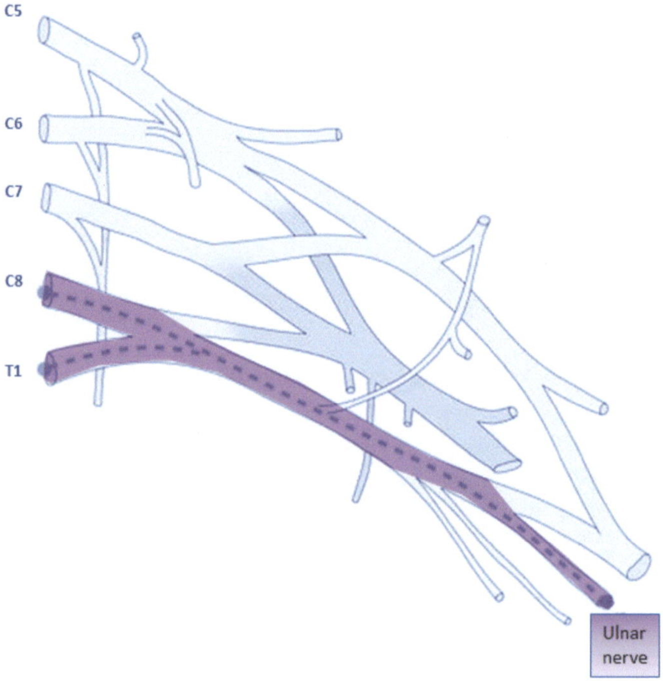

Fig. 2.1 The terminal branch of the brachial plexus

- At the wrist, the nerve passes lateral to the pisiform bone and superficial to the flexor retinaculum and enters the hand via Guyon's canal where it divides into superficial and deep branches (Fig. 2.4).

*The other four branches being the musculocutaneous, median, axillary, and radial nerves.

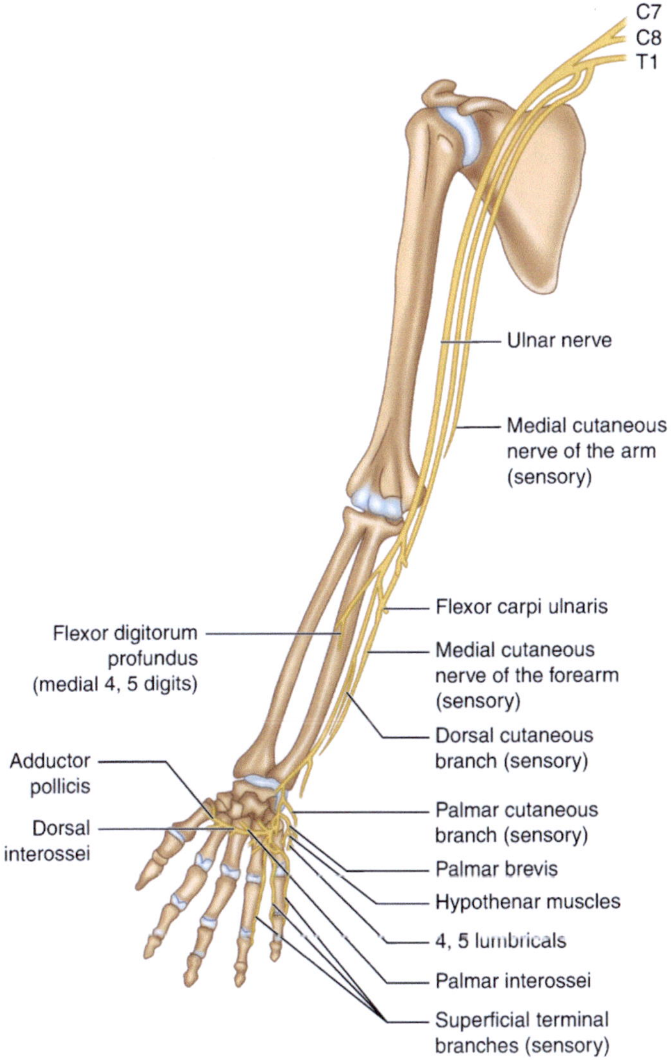

Fig. 2.2 Ulnar nerve in the arm

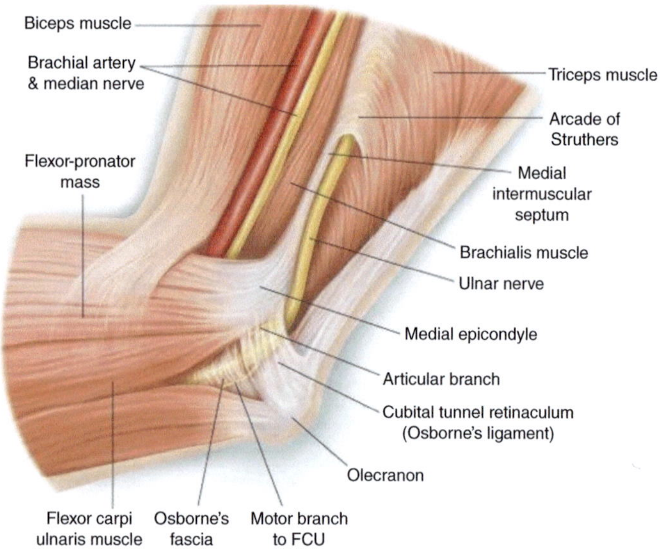

Fig. 2.3 Ulnar nerve at the elbow

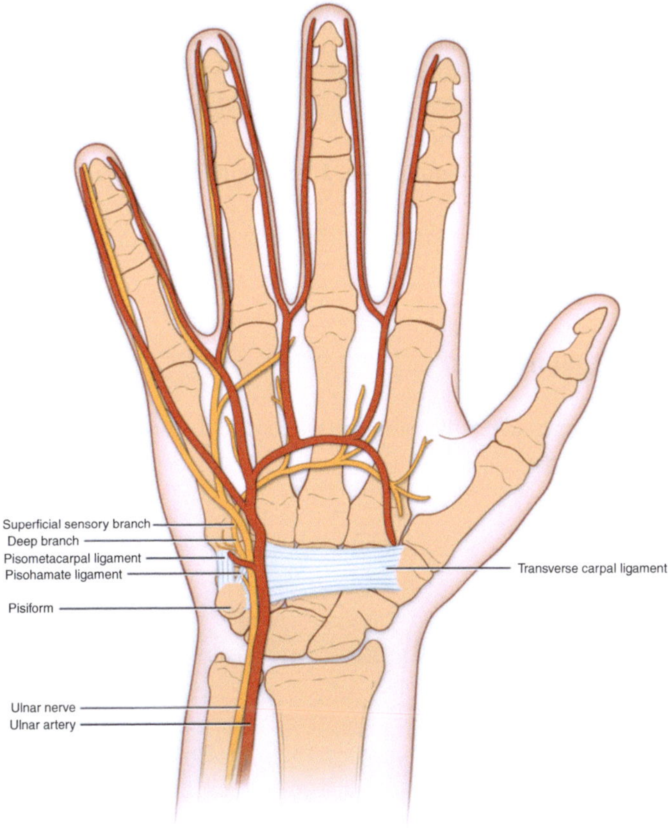

Fig. 2.4 Guyon's canal

2.2 Function

2.2.1 Motor

- Supplies flexor carpi ulnaris and the ulnar half of flexor digitorum profundus and the ulnar intrinsic muscles of the hand.

2.2.1.1 Intrinsic Function (Fig. 2.5)

- Adductors of the fingers (Fig. 2.5a): Palmar interossei
- Abductors of the fingers (Fig. 2.5b): Dorsal interossei
- Flexion at the MP joints and extension at the IP joints: (Fig. 2.5c): Lumbricals
- Adductor of the thumb: (Fig. 2.5d): Adductor policis

(Note the mnemonics for the function of the interossei: Fig. 2.5a, b)

2.2.2 Sensory

- The ulnar side of the palm and the medial one and a half fingers (Fig. 2.5e).

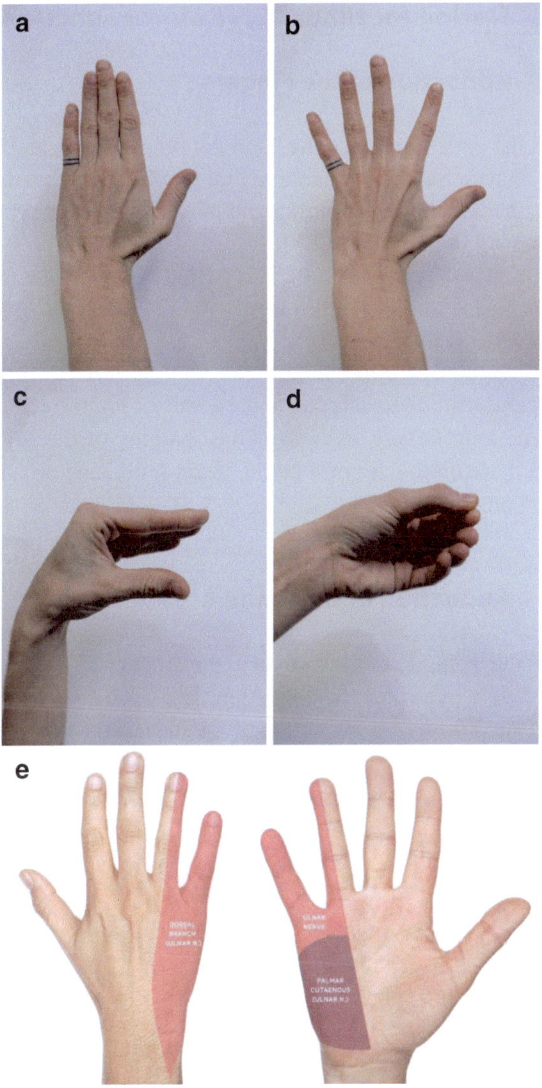

Fig. 2.5 Ulnar intrinsic function (recall the mnemonic): (**a**) Adduction of fingers; (Pad: *P*almar interossei: *ad*duct). (**b**) Abduction of fingers; (Dab: *D*orsal interossei: *ab*duct). (**c**) Flexion at the MP joints and extension at the IP joints: lumbricals. (**d**) Adduction of the thumb: Adductor policis. (**e**) Sensory innervation

2.3 Testing for Ulnar Nerve Motor Function

2.3.1 Adduction of the Fingers

- Ask the patient to place the hand flat on a surface, and adduct the fingers, trapping something thin like a card between them.
- Ask the patient to grip firmly and attempt to prevent you from removing the card (Fig. 2.6).
- If the metacarpal heads are lifted even 1 cm off the surface, there is a significant spurious increase in adductor force (see below). Test this on yourself!
- It is essential that the hand is flat on a surface, to avoid this spurious result which is due to the adductor force being exerted by the long flexors, as well as the anatomy of the MP joints which are on the arc of a circle, again producing an adductor force on flexion.

2.3.2 Abduction of the Fingers

- Get the patient to fully abduct the fingers and resist your attempt to overcome the abduction (Fig. 2.7).
- Test specifically for abduction of the index finger as this gives you the opportunity to see and palpate the bulk of the first dorsal interosseous muscle (Fig. 2.8).

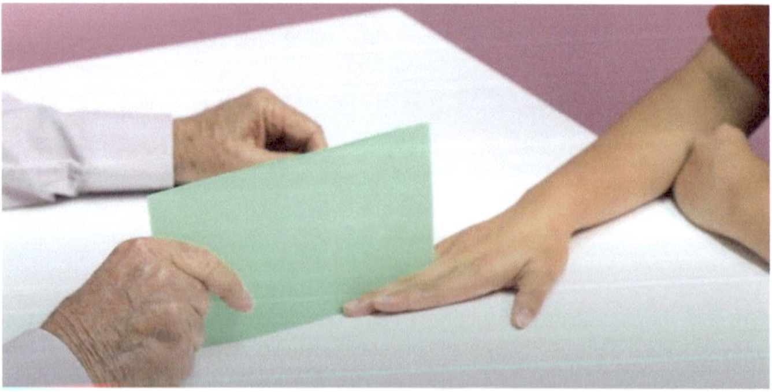

Fig. 2.6 Testing adductor function

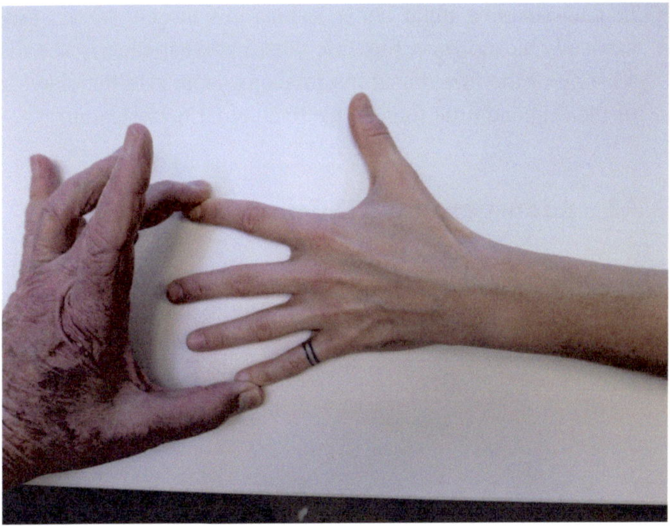

Fig. 2.7 Testing abductor function

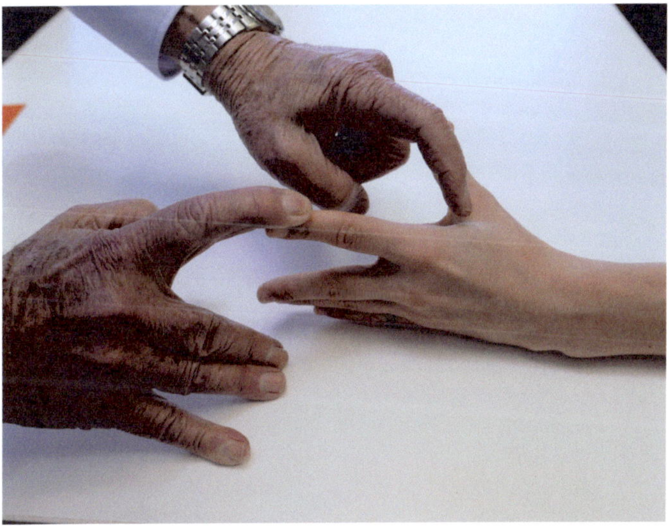

Fig. 2.8 Testing first dorsal interosseous

- In long-standing ulnar nerve lesions this muscle wastes dramatically as shown in Fig. 2.9, where you can clearly see the wasting of the first dorsal interosseous. Note also the clawing of the ring and little fingers due to an ulnar nerve lesion.

2.3.3 Adduction of the Thumb

- Adduction of the thumb is assessed by approximating the pulp of the thumb to the radial side of the index finger as in the key grip.

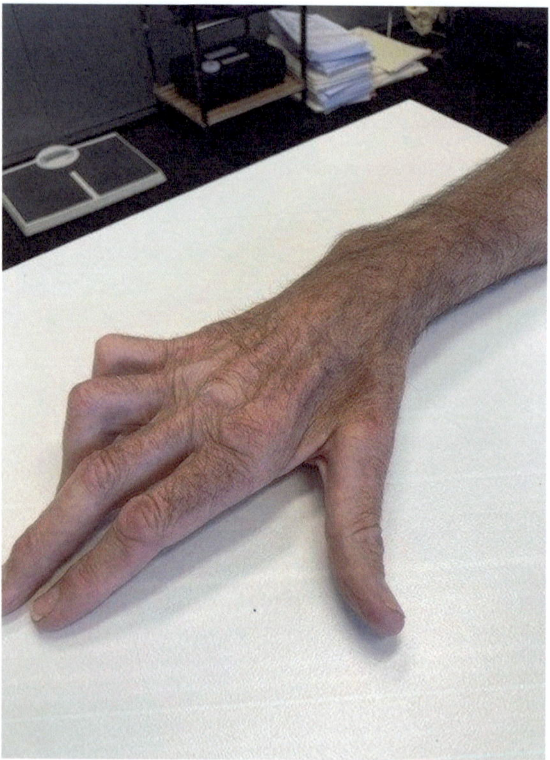

Fig. 2.9 Ulnar claw hand: wasting of first dorsal interosseous and clawing of ring and little fingers

- Ask the patient to hold firmly on to a piece of paper or card between the thumb and index finger with both hands, while you do likewise from the opposite side.
- Then ask the patient to try and prevent you from pulling the paper away.
- When there is normal function of the ulnar nerve, the patient will be able to hold the paper firmly.
- However, in an ulnar nerve lesion, when the function of adductor pollicis is weak or absent, the patient will attempt to hold the paper using the long flexor of the thumb, resulting in marked flexion at the IP joint (Fig. 2.10). This is known as a positive Froment's sign.
- It is worth noting that in testing for adduction of the thumb in a normal hand, you will see that the IP joint of the thumb is held in slight flexion (Fig. 2.11). Test this on yourself. This is due to the action of flexor pollicis longus (FPL). If this did not happen, the IP joint of the thumb would simply go into hyper-extension. The long flexor therefore stabilises the IP joint, working in conjunction with adductor pollicis, to give maximal power.

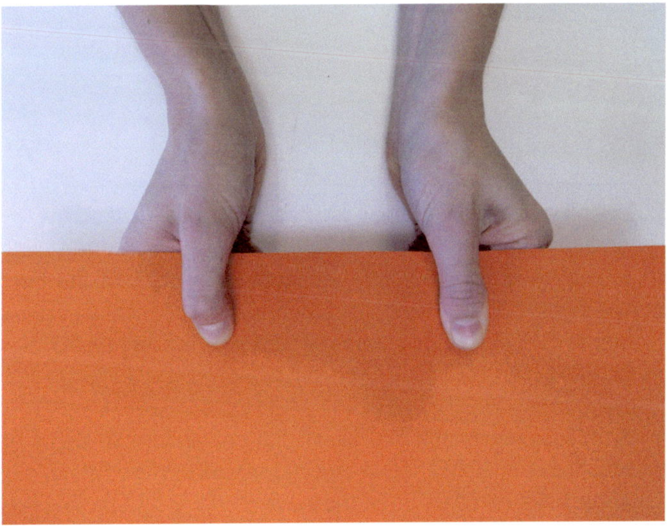

Fig. 2.10 Positive Froment's sign on the patient's right

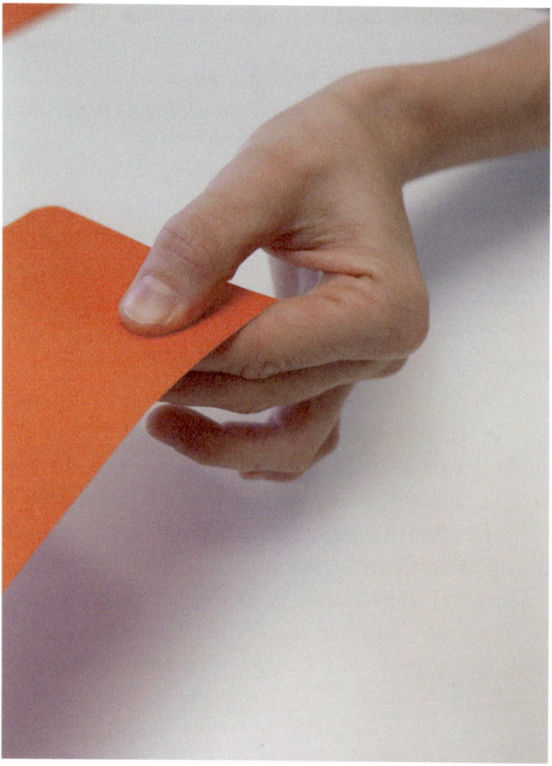

Fig. 2.11 Flexion of IP joint of thumb with adduction

2.4 Testing for Ulnar Nerve Sensory Function

(It is helpful to consider here the sensory function of the three nerves that supply the hand, the radial, ulnar. and medial nerves).

Figure 2.12 shows the commonly accepted sensory innervation of the hand.

- The ulnar nerve supplies the medial one and a half digits on both the palmar and dorsal aspects, as well as the adjacent part of the palm and dorsum of the hand.
- The median supplies the rest of the palmar aspect of the hand and supplies the dorsum of the distal part of the lateral three

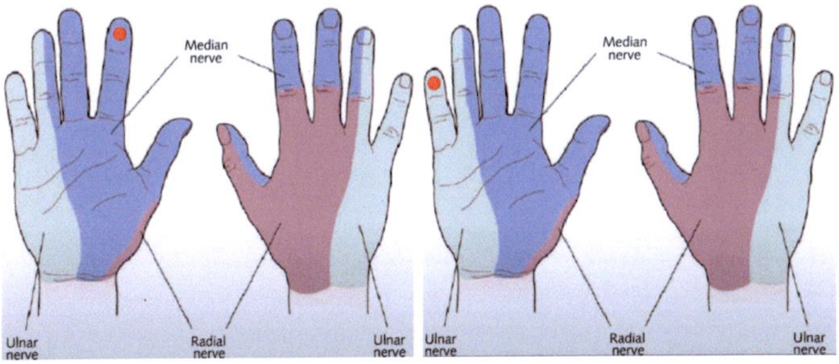

Fig. 2.12 Front of hand showing autonomous zones of median and ulnar nerves

and a half digits to a level somewhere between the DIP and PIP joints.

- The radial nerve supplies the rest of the dorsum of the hand.
- Despite the description provided above, there is some overlap of the sensory regions. It is therefore important to note that there are also so-called autonomous zones which are those areas very specifically supplied by a particular nerve.
- For the median nerve, this is the pulp of the index finger; for the ulnar nerve, this is the pulp of the little finger (Fig. 2.12); and for the radial nerve, it is the web space on the dorsum of the hand between the thumb and index finger (Fig. 2.13).

As with sensory testing in general, this needs to be carried out slowly and deliberately. The patient needs to understand what you are doing and needs enough time to consider and respond. Sensory testing needs to be repeated and always compared to the other side.

My preference is to use a K-wire (Kirschner wire) with a bent end so that it does not roll away and the sharp end not sharp enough to penetrate the skin and draw blood (Fig. 2.14).

Note: In assessing impairment according to AMA5, the extent of sensory loss is determined using two-point discrimination (AMA Guides to the Evaluation of Permanent Impairment, Fifth Edition, page 447, Table 16-5).

How is sensation in the hand tested in a patient who is unconscious or a child who is too young to understand? Here are three suggestions:

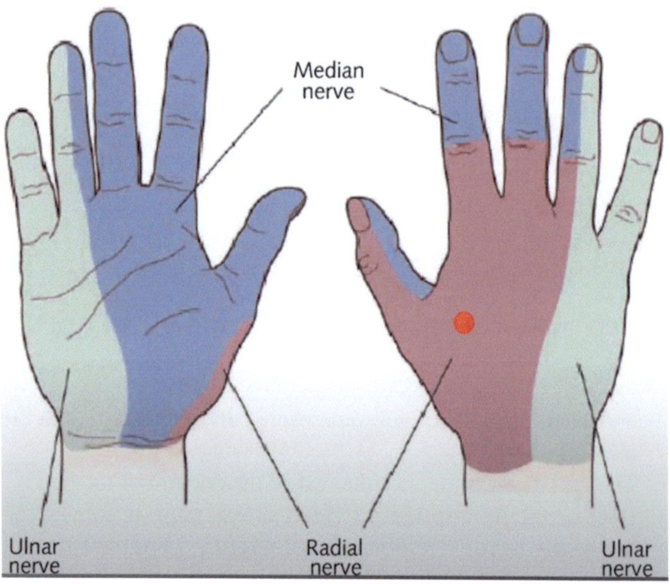

Fig. 2.13 Back of hand showing autonomous zone for radial nerve

- With nerve damage there is loss of autonomic supply of the fingers and loss of sudomotor function (sweating). As a result, the pulp of the affected digit or digits feels dry when compared to the unaffected fingers. Telling the difference requires careful examination and practice!
- The so-called 'violin test' is carried out by running a smooth plastic object such as a pen over the digit. With normal sensation and therefore normal sweating, running a smooth object over the digit is associated with a feeling of slight resistance because of the moisture (Fig. 2.15). When sensation is lost and the skin is dry (due to lack of sweating), there is much less resistance. This can be illustrated by on one's own normal finger and then repeating the test after placing a piece of tissue paper between the digit and the pen (Fig. 2.16).

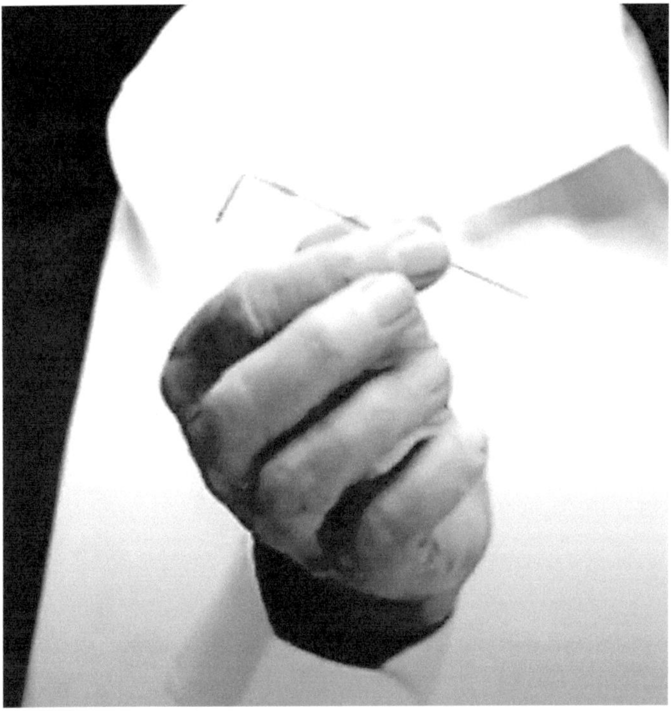

Fig. 2.14 K-wire

- The 'prune test': If you have spent a lot of time in water, particularly warm water, you will notice how the skin of the pulp of the fingers tends to wrinkle (Fig. 2.17). This does not happen in denervated digits. The mechanism is thought to be due to vasoconstriction, and there is much discussion as to the evolutionary reason for this.

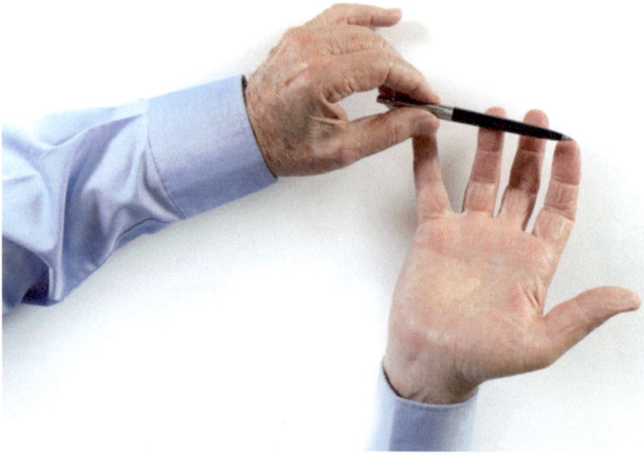

Fig. 2.15 Violin test

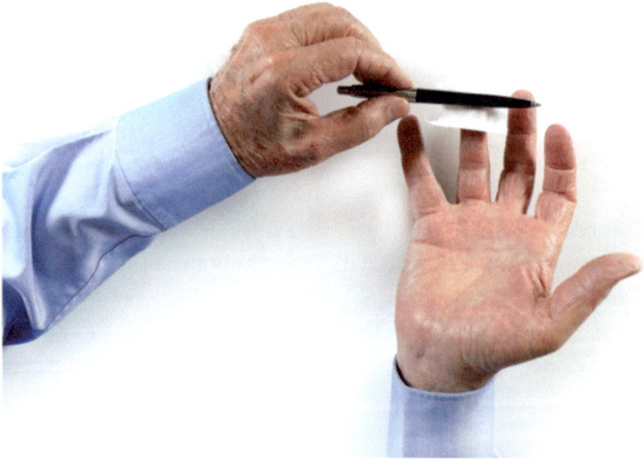

Fig. 2.16 Violin test with tissue paper

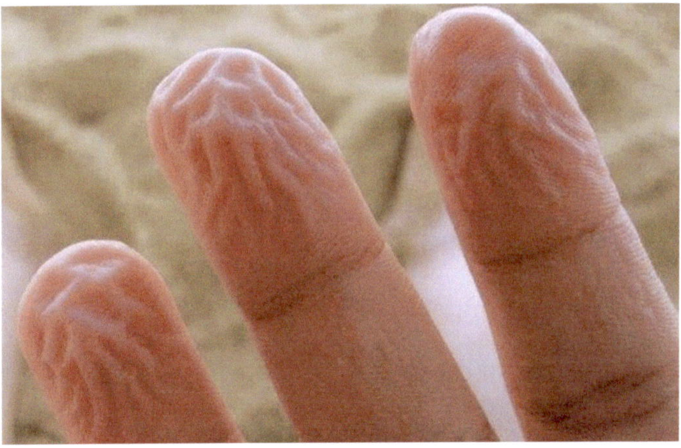

Fig. 2.17 Prune test

2.5 Lesions of the Ulnar Nerve

2.5.1 Cubital Tunnel Syndrome

- This condition is due to compression of the ulnar nerve in the cubital tunnel or related structures on the medial side of the elbow. This is the most common site of entrapment/compression of the nerve.

2.5.1.1 Symptoms

- Numbness and paraesthesias in the little finger and ulnar half of the ring finger.
- The symptoms occur either spontaneously or can are associated with prolonged elbow flexion such as when using a mobile phone, or with pressure on the medial aspect of the elbow on a firm surface, for example, long-distance driving with the elbow resting on the arm rest.
- There may be weakness of the ulnar nerve innervated intrinsic muscles of the hand.

2.5.1.2 Physical Signs

- Positive Tinel's sign (tapping over the ulnar nerve on the posteromedial aspect of the elbow associated with complaint of parasthesias in the ulnar nerve distribution).
- Weakness or wasting of the intrinsic muscles supplied by the ulnar nerve.
- Severe cases may develop an ulnar claw hand.

2.5.2 Ulnar Tunnel Syndrome (Guyon's Canal)

- Compression of the distal ulnar nerve at the level of the wrist as it enters the hand via Guyon's canal*, where the nerve divides into superficial sensory and deep motor branches (An uncommon condition)
- Physical signs will depend on the site of compression within the canal giving either:
- Combined motor and sensory loss
- Sensory loss only
- Motor loss only
- Differs from cubital tunnel syndrome:
  - Tinel's sign positive at the wrist rather than the elbow.
  - Normal sensation on the dorsum of the hand (the dorsal cutaneous branch winds around the distal ulna proximal to Guyon's canal*, and is therefore spared in distal but not proximal lesions)
  - No involvement of ulnar extrinsic muscles

2.5.2.1 *Guyon's Canal: Anatomical Boundaries

- Extends from the level of the pisiform to the hamate—approximately 4 cm in length (Fig. 2.18)
- Borders:
  - Floor—flexor retinaculum
  - Roof—palmar carpal ligament
  - Medial (ulnar)—pisiform, abductor digiti minimi muscle
  - Lateral (radial)—hook of hamate

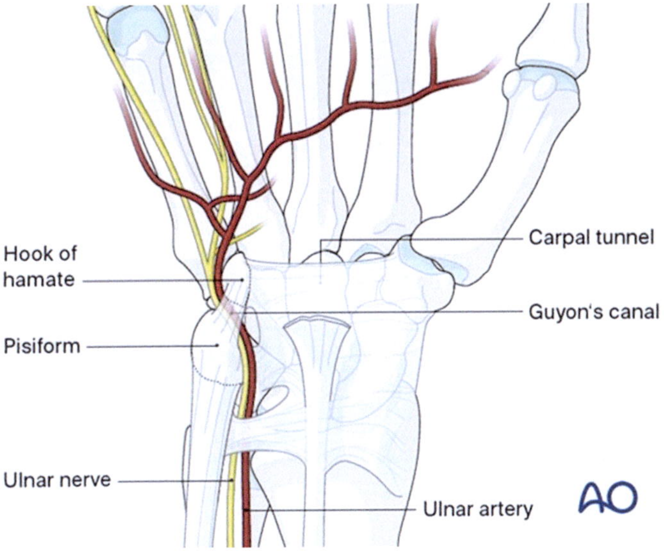

Fig. 2.18 Guyon's canal—anatomical boundaries

2.6 Ulnar Claw Hand

2.6.1 An Explanation of the Deformity

Figure 2.19 shows the typical deformity in an ulnar claw hand, with extension at the level of the MP joints and flexion at both the PIP and DIP joints of the ring and little fingers.

The explanation of this deformity is very instructive and satisfying. However, two different issues need to be understood in this regard. The first is the difference between balanced and unbalanced paralysis, and the second is an understanding of the function of the intrinsic muscles of the hand.

1. *The difference between balanced and unbalanced paralysis (using the radial nerve as an example)*

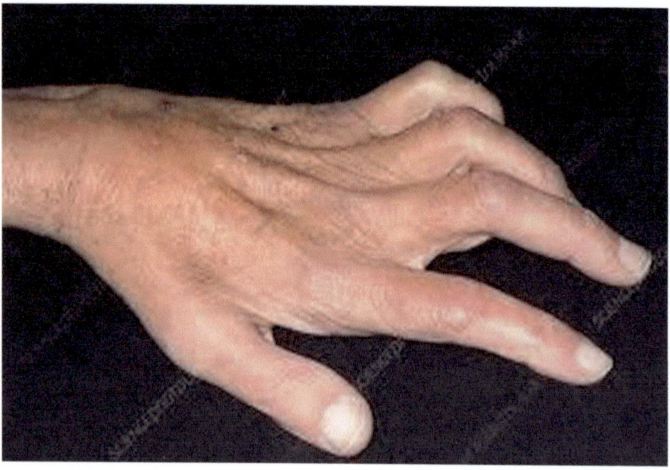

Fig. 2.19 Ulnar claw hand

- Say, for example, a person has a complete lesion of the radial nerve in the upper arm which does not recover.
- This leads to loss of extensor function of the wrist with resultant wrist drop and eventual deformity due to the unopposed action of the wrist flexors.
- This is an unbalanced paralysis, which leads to deformity.
- Now assume a person has a brachial plexus lesion with loss of both flexor and extensor function of the wrist.
- This is a balanced paralysis which leads to flailness.
- An unbalanced paralysis therefore leads to deformity; a balanced paralysis leads to flailness.

It is worth noting that the treatment for each of these conditions is very different. (Please note that these are general surgical/orthopaedic principles which would apply to any similar situation).

- If one has an unbalanced paralysis of the wrist due to paralysis of the extensor muscles, with a still mobile deformity, the treatment is to transfer one of the flexor tendons of the wrist to the extensor tendons, to give some extensor function and therefore restore balance.

- On the other hand, if one has a balanced paralysis due to paralysis of the flexor and extensor muscles which leads to flailness, the treatment is stabilisation, either externally by means of a splint, or internally by fusion of the wrist.

Condition	Outcome	Treatment
Unbalanced paralysis →	Deformity →	Tendon transfer
Balanced paralysis →	Flailness →	Stabilisation—(External/internal)

2. *Intrinsic muscle function*
   - The second issue or principle to understand is the function of the intrinsic muscles of the hand.
   - Figure 2.20 shows that contraction of the intrinsic muscles causes flexion at the MP joints and extension at the IP joints.
   - It is important to realise that the long flexors do not have any direct effect on the MP joints, and that flexion of these joints follows flexion of the DIP and PIP joints in a 'roll-up' action.

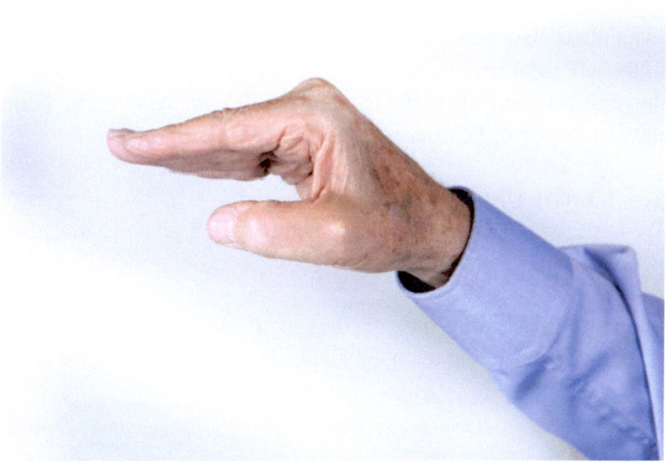

Fig. 2.20 Intrinsic function: flexion MP extension IP

- Therefore, when the fingers are extended there can be no 'roll-up' action, and the only way one can flex the MP joints is via the intrinsics.

2.6.2 Explanation of the Ulnar Claw Hand Deformity[1]

- Note again the deformity in an ulnar claw hand, with extension or hyper-extension at the level of the MP joints and flexion at the IP joints of the ring and little fingers.
- Concentrating first on the MP joints and recall that the intrinsics cause flexion of these joints. In an ulnar nerve lesion with loss of function of the intrinsics, there is loss of flexion of the MP joints, while there is still active (unbalanced) extension.
- So, one has an unbalanced paralysis which leads to deformity in favour of extension.
- At the level of the IP joints, the long flexors are still functioning, whereas the extensors (that is the intrinsics) are not functioning, leading to a deformity in favour of flexion.

2.6.3 Summary

In an ulnar claw hand, there is an unbalanced paralysis at the level of the MP joint leading to deformity in favour of extension and an unbalanced paralysis at the level of the IP joints leading to deformity in favour of flexion.

2.6.3.1 The Ulnar Paradox

We need to consider the difference between a high and a low ulnar nerve lesion.

- In the low lesion, the function of the long flexor tendons is preserved, leading to an unbalanced paralysis at the level of the

[1]Roger Pillemer, "*Handbook of Upper Extremity Examination*" Springer 2022. Chapter 4, Pages 76–79.

IP joints, which in turn leads to deformity in favour of flexion as noted above.

- However, in a high ulnar nerve lesion, the long flexors of the little and ring fingers lose their nerve supply (FDP), and therefore instead of an unbalanced paralysis at the DIP joint in favour of flexion, there is a balanced paralysis which leads to flailness rather than deformity.
- The deformity is therefore less noticeable.

Hence the use of the term 'paradox'. The high ulnar nerve lesion results in less deformity than a low lesion, whereas one would normally expect the opposite.

Examination of the Hand 3

In my previous book *Handbook of Upper Extremity Examination*,[1] I have dealt with the examination of the hand under three headings:

- The anatomy and function of the hand
- The systematic examination of the hand
- An examination of specific conditions relating to the hand

What I would like to do in this chapter is to describe the physical signs that we look for and elicit in our examination of the hand. This will include the various tests and signs described in the chapters in this book on the median and ulnar nerves.

3.1 Neurological

Three nerves supply the motor and sensory function of the hand, namely, the median, ulnar, and radial nerves. Note that the median and ulnar nerves supply extrinsic and intrinsic muscles, whereas the radial nerve supplies only extrinsic muscles.

[1] *Handbook of Upper Extremity Examination. A Practical Guide*. Springer 2022.

R. Pillemer, *Physical Signs in Orthopedic and Neurologic Disorders*, https://doi.org/10.1007/978-3-031-99529-3_3

3.1.1 Motor Function

Three tests for each nerve:

3.1.1.1 Median Nerve

1. Abduction of thumb (Fig. 3.1)
2. Opposition of thumb (Fig. 3.2)
3. Thenar eminence (Fig. 3.3)

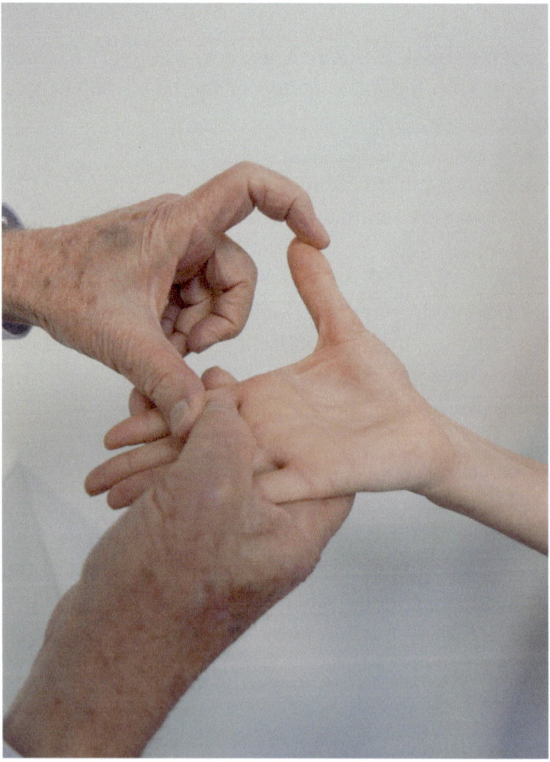

Fig. 3.1 Abduction of the thumb

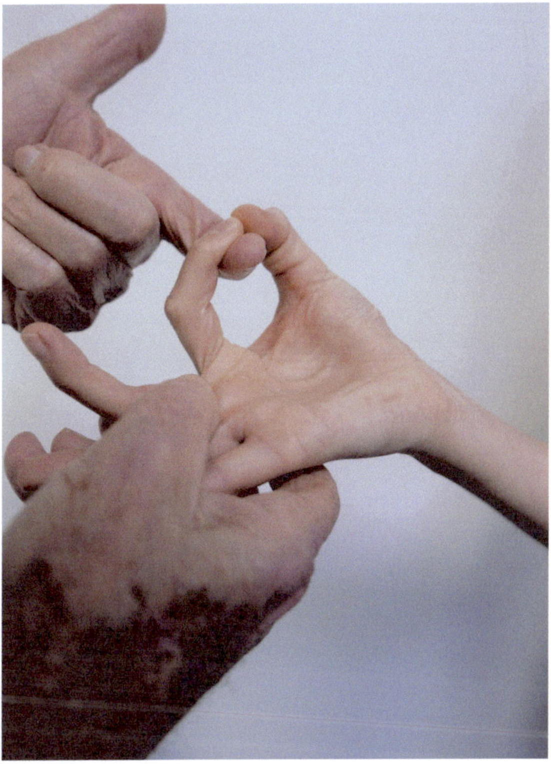

Fig. 3.2 Opposition of the thumb

3.1.1.2 Ulnar Nerve

1. Abduction of fingers (Fig. 3.4)
2. Adduction of fingers (Fig. 3.5)
3. Adduction of the thumb—Froment's sign (Fig. 3.6)

3.1.1.3 Radial Nerve

1. Extension of wrist (Fig. 3.7)
2. Extension of fingers (Fig. 3.8)
3. Extension of thumb (Fig. 3.9)

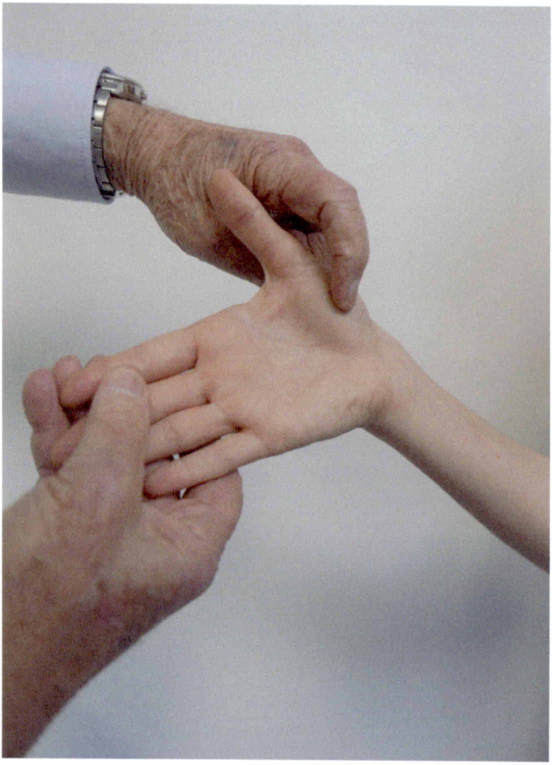

Fig. 3.3 Thenar eminence

3.1.2 Intrinsic Motor Function

Points worth noting:

- Small muscles that arise and insert in the hand.
- These control and produce all of the fine movements of the hand.
- All the intrinsic muscles that move the thumb are supplied by the median nerve, with the exception of adductor pollicis which is supplied by the ulnar nerve (Fig. 3.10)
- 'LOAF'—the intrinsic muscles supplied by the median nerve (Fig. 3.11)
  - *L*ateral two lumbricals

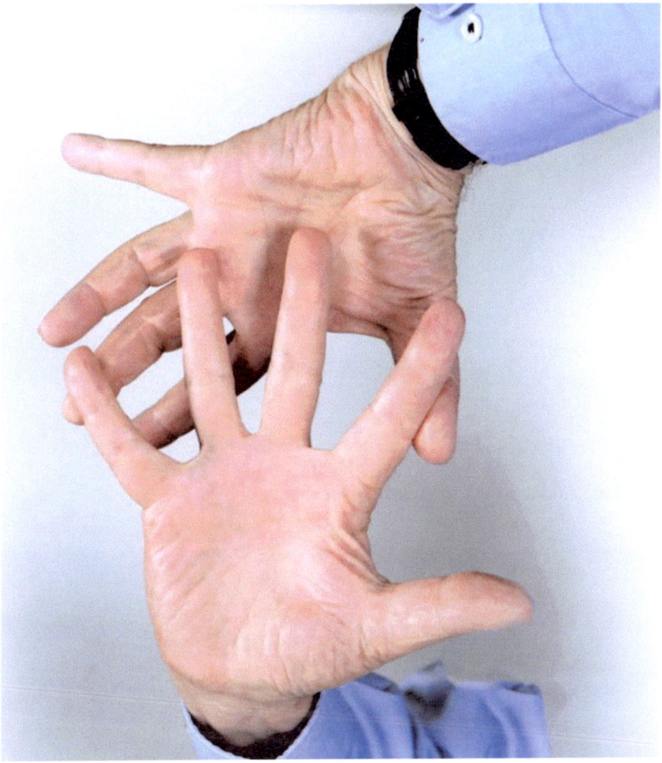

Fig. 3.4 Abduction of fingers

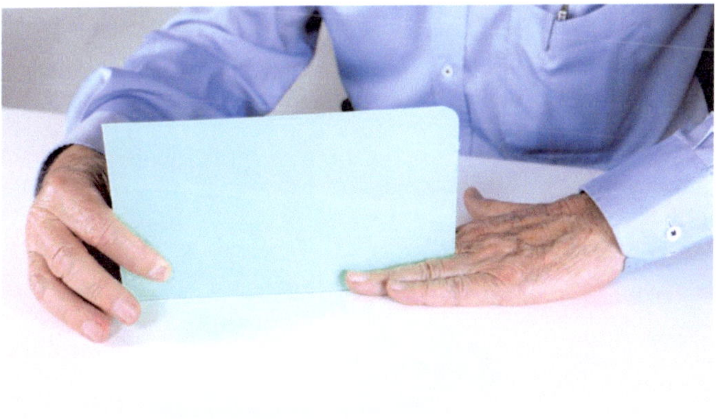

Fig. 3.5 Adduction of fingers

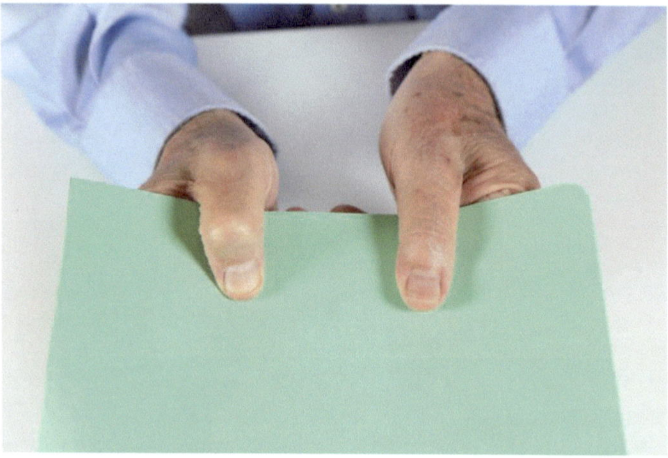

Fig. 3.6 Adduction of the thumb—Froment's sign

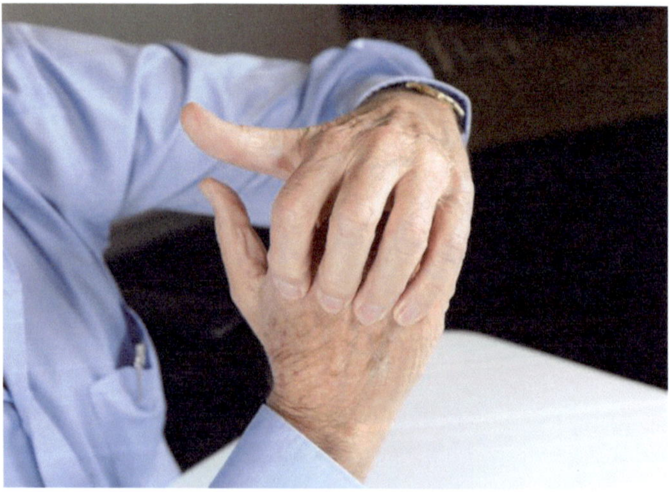

Fig. 3.7 Extension of the wrist

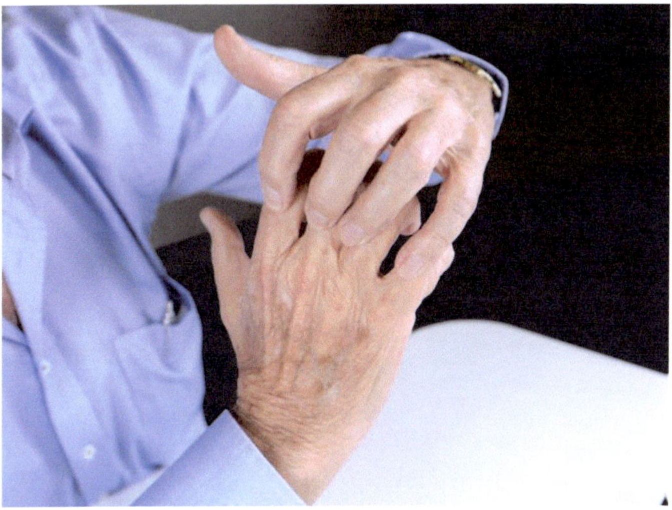

Fig. 3.8 Extension of the fingers

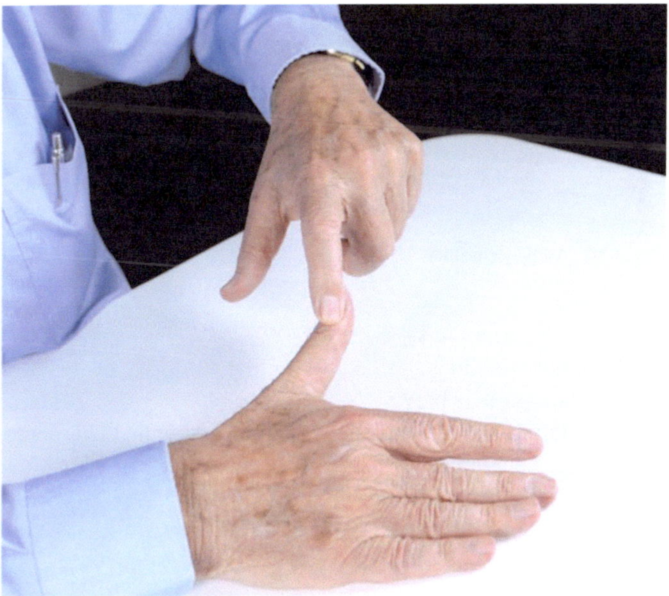

Fig. 3.9 Extension of the thumb

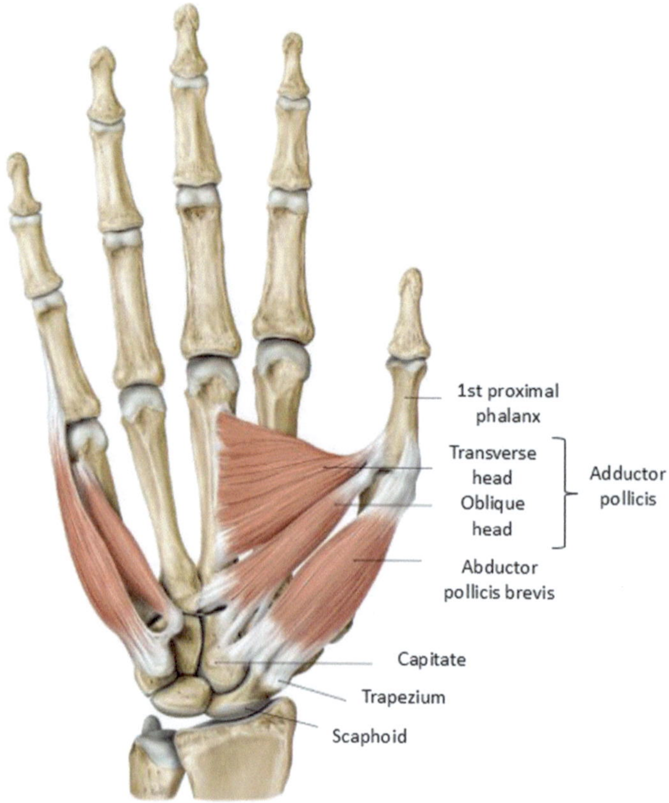

Fig. 3.10 Adductor pollicis

  - *O*pponens pollicis
  - *A*bductor pollicis
  - *F*lexor pollicis brevis
- All of the rest of the intrinsics are supplied by the ulnar nerve.
  - Hypothenar muscles
  - Medial two lumbricals
  - Adductor pollicis
  - Palmaris brevis
  - Interossei of the hand

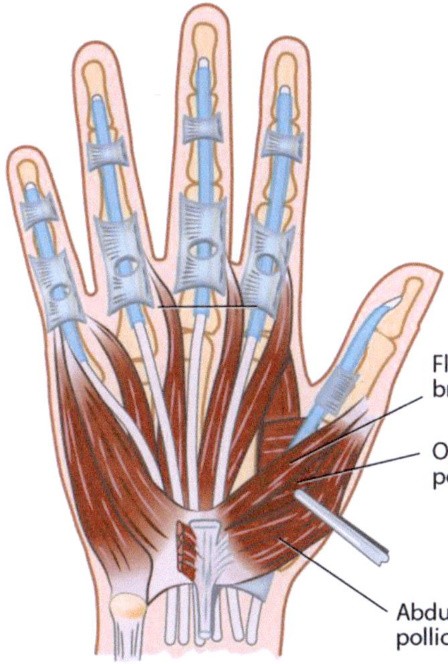

Fig. 3.11 Median nerve intrinsics

Recall the mnemonic:

Pad: *p*almar interosseous, a*d*duct.
Dab: *d*orsal interosseous, a*b*duct.

3.1.3 Extrinsic Motor Function

- Extension of the wrist, fingers, and thumb are described above, all supplied by the radial nerve.
- Flexion of the fingers is carried out by the long flexor tendons, flexor digitorum profundus (FDP) which attaches to the base of the distal phalanx and enables flexion at the DIP joint, and flexor digitorum superficialis (FDS) which attaches to the middle phalanx and enables flexion at the PIP joint (Fig. 3.12).

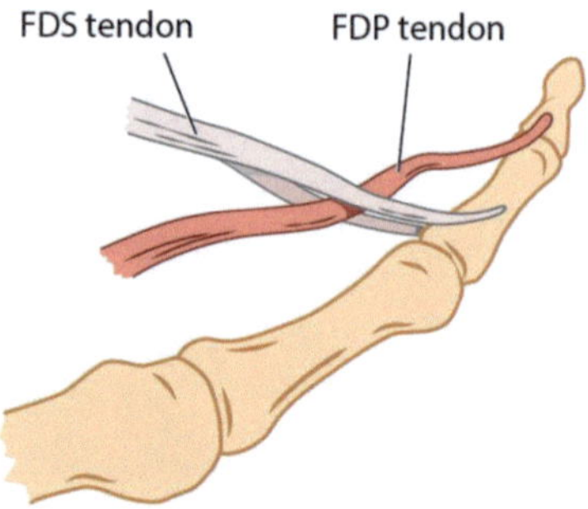

Fig. 3.12 The superficialis tendon splits before inserting into the middle phalanx

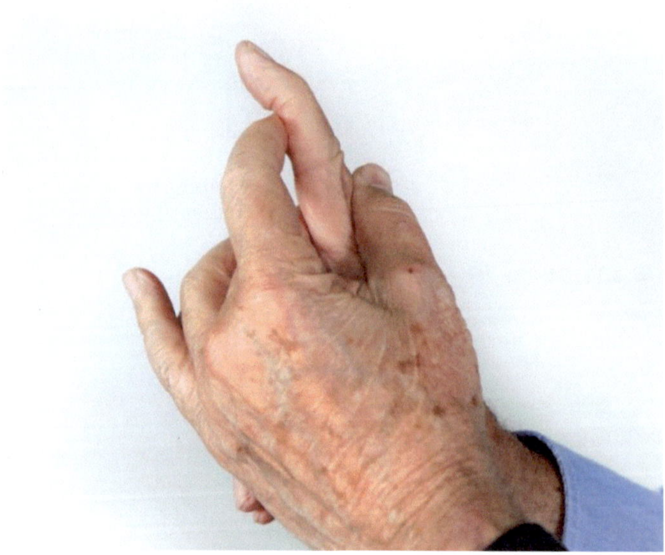

Fig. 3.13 Testing for flexor digitorum profundus (FDP)

- To isolate the function of FDP, keep the MP and PIP joints in extension and the flexion that occurs at the DIP joint in due to FDP only (Fig. 3.13).
- To isolate FDS, hold three of the four fingers and flex the remaining finger. All flexion now occurs at the PIP joint and is due to FDS only (Fig. 3.14). Test each finger in turn.

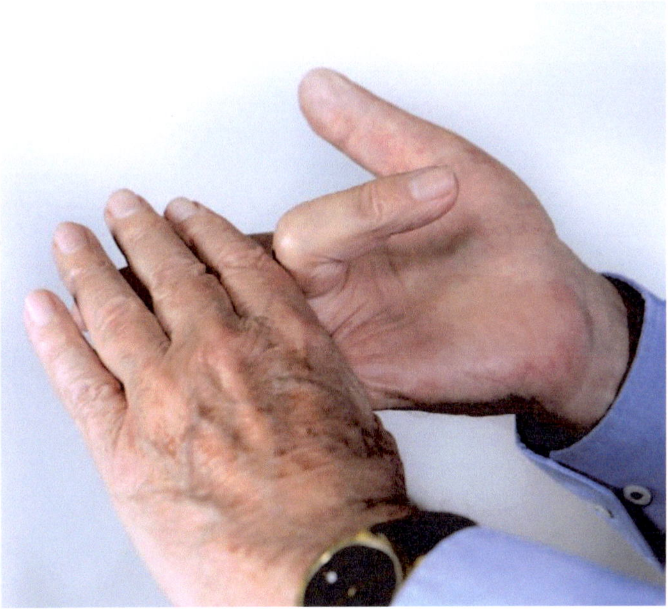

Fig. 3.14 Testing for flexor digitorum superficialis (FDS)

- Flexor pollicis longus (FPL) to the thumb is tested in a similar fashion (Fig. 3.15).

Note that the median nerve supplies all of FDS as well as FDP to the index and middle fingers, while the ulnar nerve supplies FDP to the ring and little fingers.

3.1.4 Sensory Function

The sensory distribution of the three nerves supplying the hand is shown in Fig. 3.16, which also shows the 'autonomous zones', being the pulp of the index finger for the median nerve, the pulp of the little finger for the ulnar nerve, and the first web space for the radial nerve.

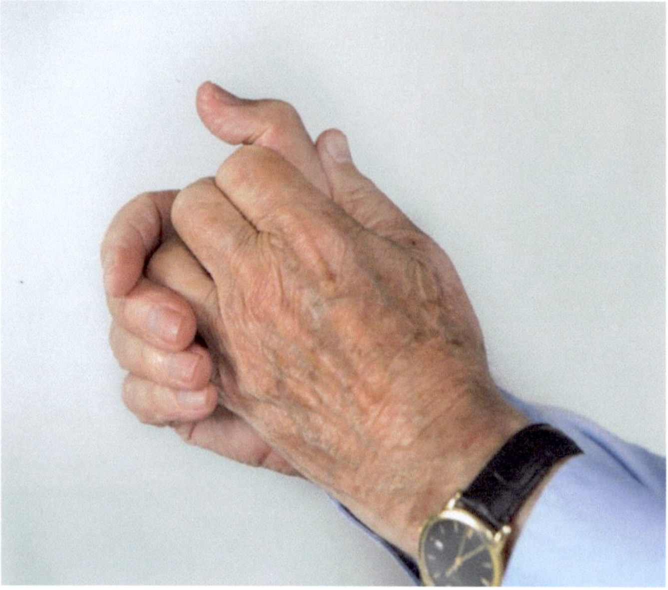

Fig. 3.15 Testing for flexor pollicis longus (FPL)

3.1.5 Screening Test

Twenty second screening test for motor and sensory function of all three nerves supplying the hand. Each nerve supplies at least one motor function test in relation to the thumb:

- Abduction for the median nerve (Fig. 3.1)
- Adduction for the ulnar nerve (Fig. 3.6)
- Extension for the radial nerve (Fig. 3.9)

Then test for the three autonomous sensory zones, and the screening test is complete!

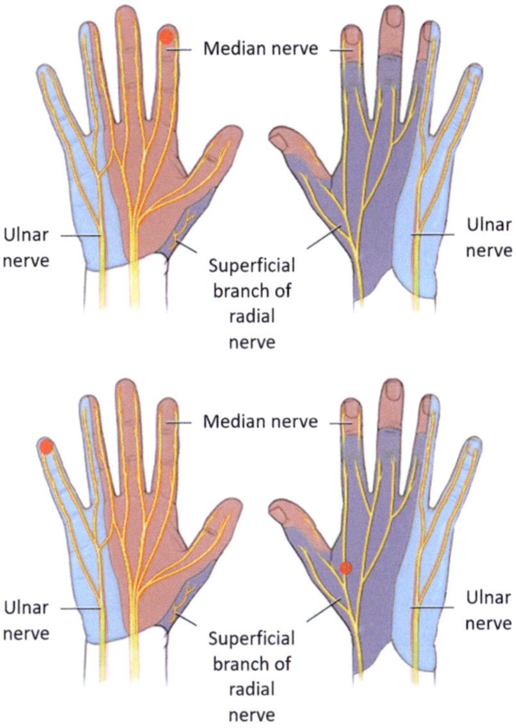

Fig. 3.16 Sensory innervation of the hand including autonomous zones

3.1.6 Sensory Testing in an Unconscious Patient or a Child Too Young to Understand

Here are three suggestions:

- The pulp of the affected digit feels dry compared to unaffected fingers. This is because with nerve damage there is loss of autonomic supply to the finger and loss of sudomotor function (sweating).
- The 'violin test' (Fig. 3.17). Running a smooth plastic object, such as a pen, over the pulp of the finger gives less resistance than over a normal finger, as a result of the dryness due to the loss of sweating noted above

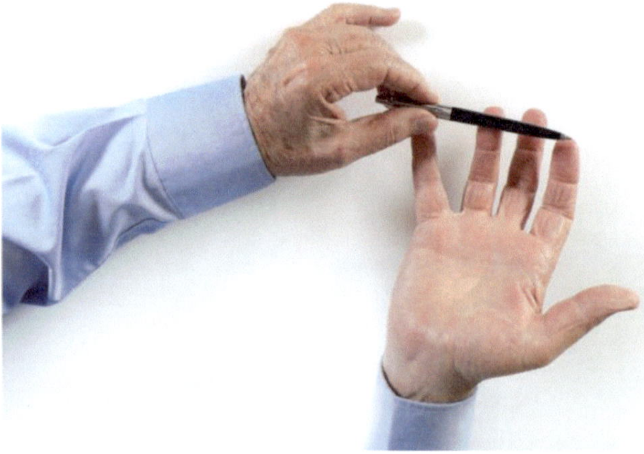

Fig. 3.17 Violin test

- The 'prune test' (Fig. 3.18). Fingers immersed in water for an extended period become wrinkled. This does not happen in denervated fingers.

3.1.7 Testing for Vascular Function: The Allen Test

The blood supply of the hand is via the radial and ulnar arteries, and Allen's test will demonstrate the patency of these vessels.

- Occlude both radial and ulnar arteries (Fig. 3.19).
- Get the patient to open and close the fingers firmly three or four times and then leave the fingers open. The hand will be seen to have blanched (Fig. 3.20).
- Release the radial artery and note how the hand perfuses.
- Repeat the test from the beginning, but now release the ulnar artery and confirm the perfusion.

The following physical signs are discussed in the chapter on the median nerve (See Sects. 1.4–1.6, pages 14–28).

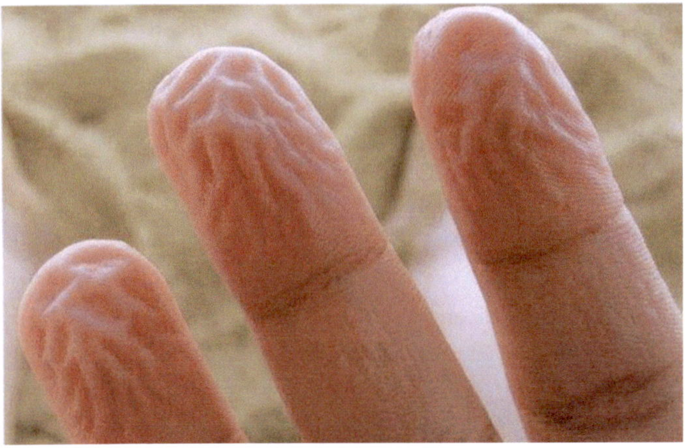

Fig. 3.18 Prune test

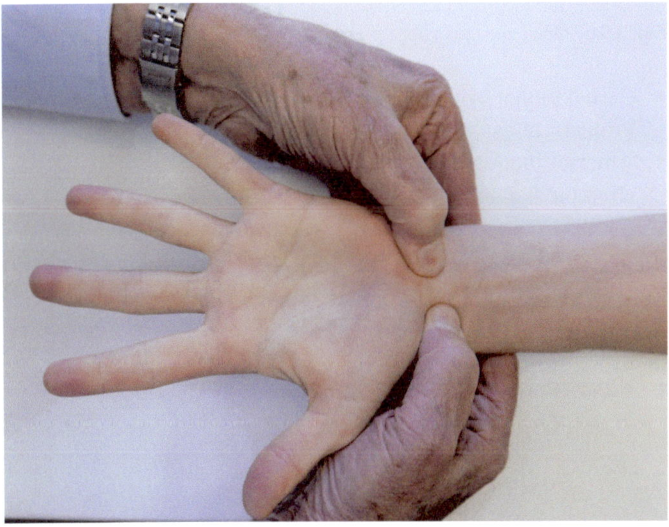

Fig. 3.19 Occlude both arteries

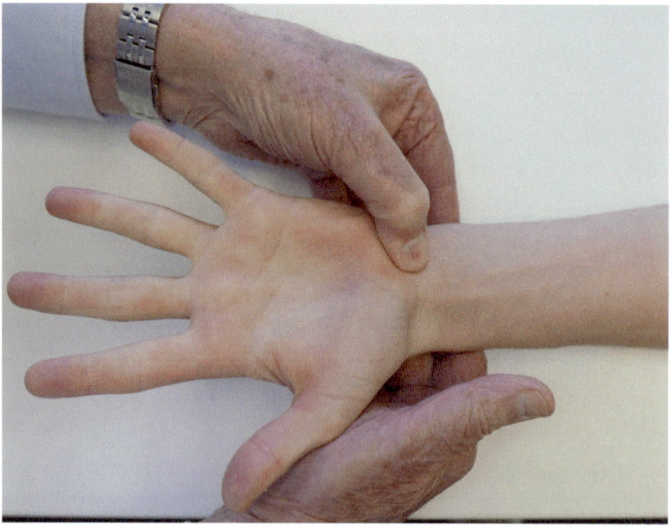

Fig. 3.20 Open and close blanch

- Carpal tunnel syndrome
- Pronator teres syndrome
- Anterior interosseous syndrome—the 'OK' sign
- High median nerve lesions—the 'Benediction sign'

The following physical signs are discussed in the chapter on the ulnar nerve (See Sects. 2.3.3, 2.4, 2.5, pages 38–47).

- Cubital tunnel syndrome
- Ulnar claw hand

3.2 DeQuervain's Tenosynovitis

- Swelling of the tendons or narrowing of the tunnel of the first dorsal extensor compartment [Extensor pollicis brevis (EPB) and abductor pollicis longus (APL) on the radial side of the distal radius] (Fig. 3.21).

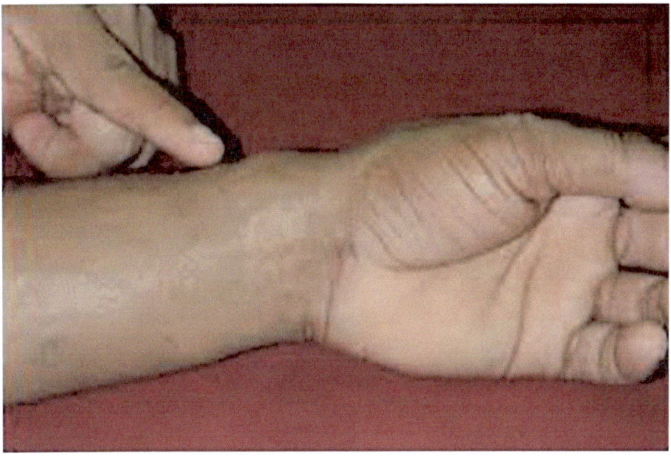

Fig. 3.21 DeQuervain's swelling

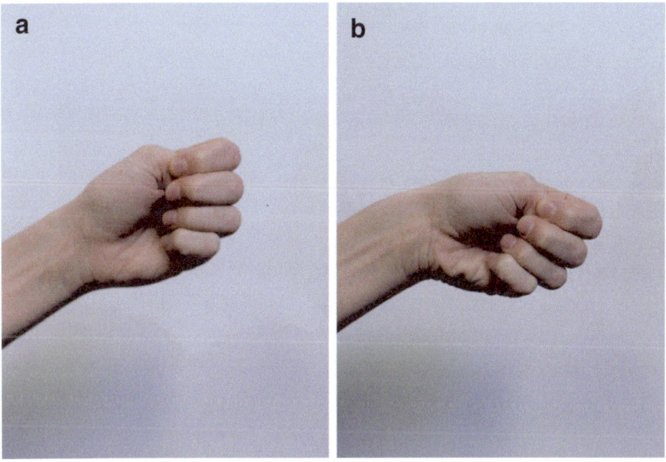

Fig. 3.22 Finkelstein's test. (**a**) neutral position. (**b**) ulnar position

- Positive Finkelstein's test: Ask the patient to hold the thumb in the palm and make a fist (Fig. 3.22). Ulnar deviation of the wrist will reproduce the pain.

3.3 Lateral Epicondylitis (Tennis Elbow)

- Localised tenderness over the lateral epicondylar region (Fig. 3.23)
- Reproduction of pain on resisted extension of the wrist with the elbow in extension (Fig. 3.24)
- Reproduction of pain on resisted extension of the middle finger with the elbow in extension (Fig. 3.25)

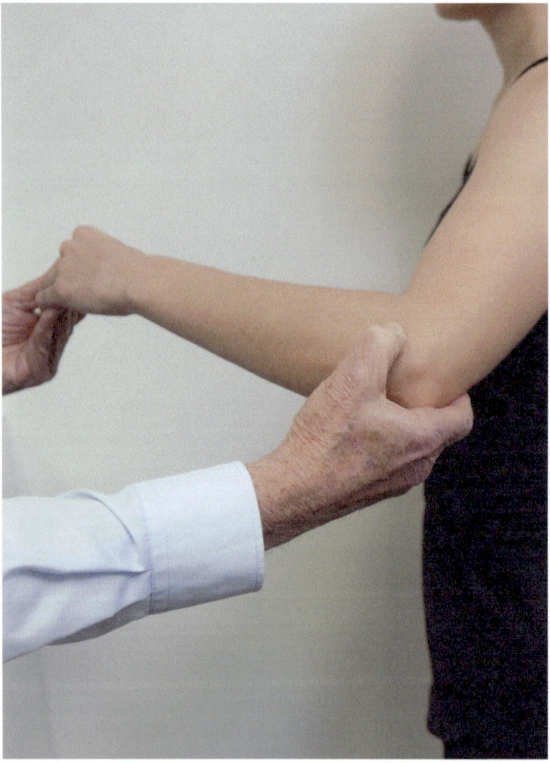

Fig. 3.23 Localised tenderness over lateral epicondyle

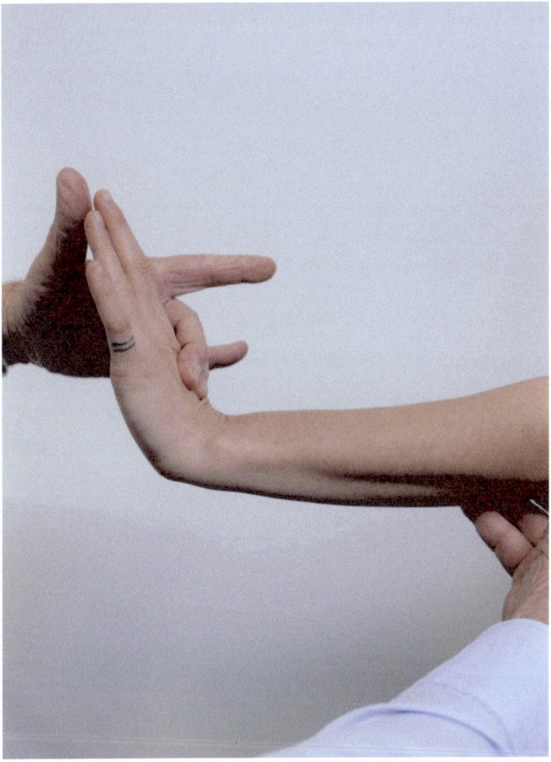

Fig. 3.24 Resisted extension of the wrist

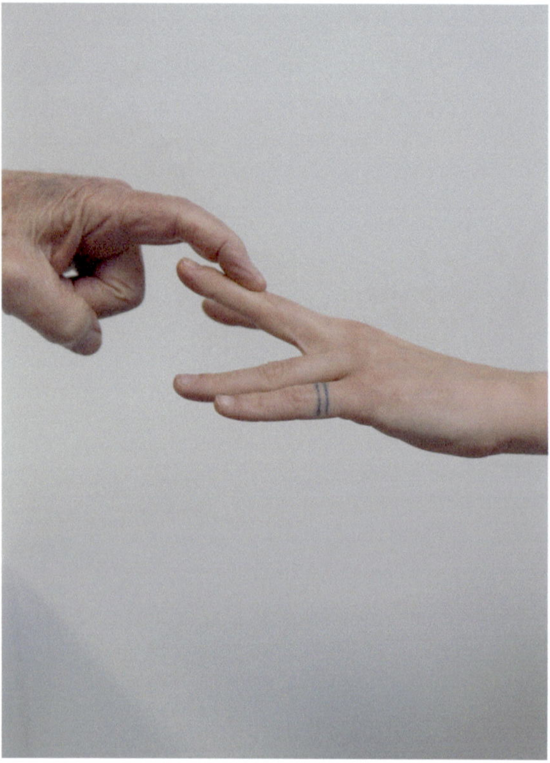

Fig. 3.25 Resisted extension of the middle finger

3.4 Boutonniere Deformity

- Injury to the insertion of the extensor tendon into the base of the middle phalanx
- Fixed flexion deformity at the PIP joint and fixed extension at the DIP joint (Fig. 3.26)

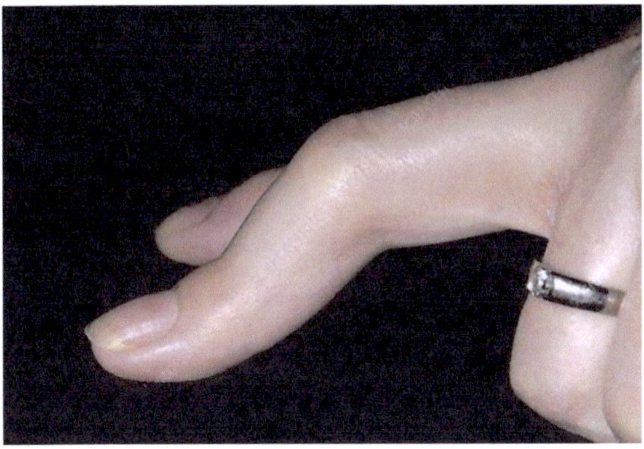

Fig. 3.26 Boutonniere deformity

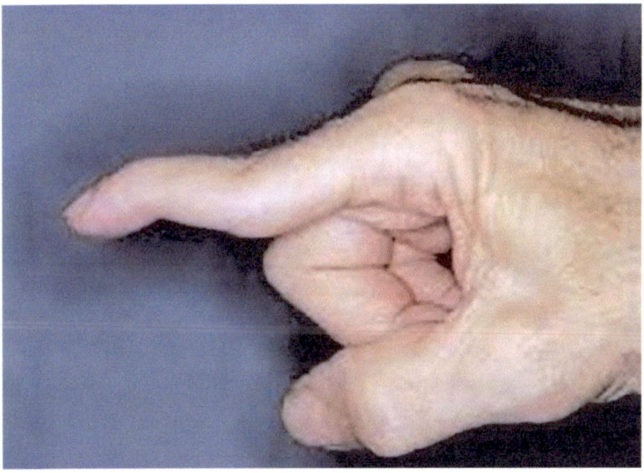

Fig. 3.27 Swan neck deformity

3.5 Swan Neck Deformity

- Hyper-extension at the PIP joint of the finger due to laxity of the volar plate (Fig. 3.27)

3.6 Mallet Finger

- Traumatic disruption of the extensor tendon into the base of the distal phalanx with either tendon rupture or avulsion of a piece of bone, with inability to actively extend the DIP joint and obvious flexion deformity (Fig. 3.28)

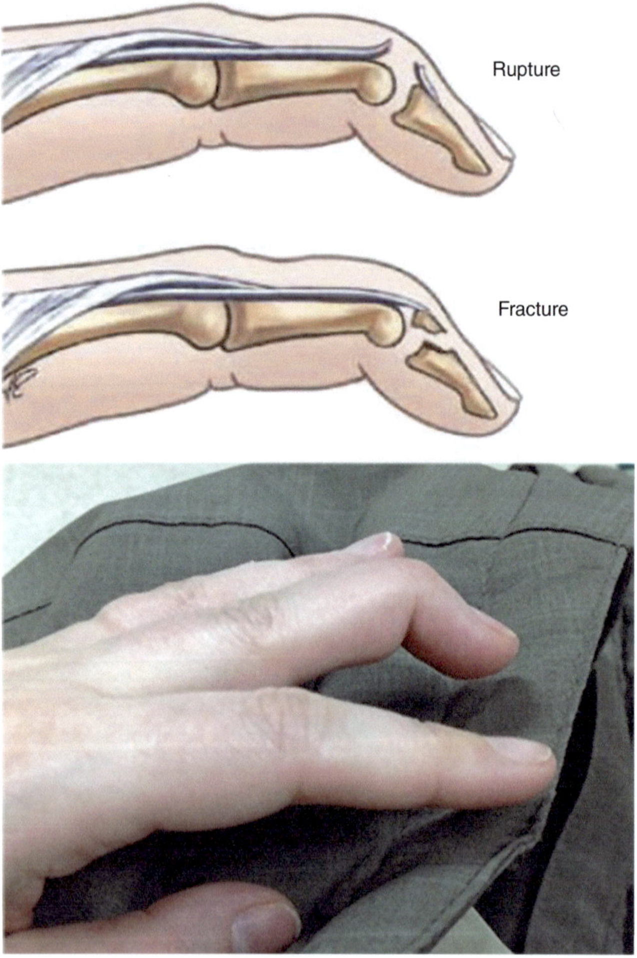

Fig. 3.28 Mallet finger deformity

3.7 Scapholunate Instability

- Damage to the scapholunate ligament can lead to a gap between the scaphoid and the lunate seen on X-ray (Fig. 3.29)
- This can lead to scapholunate advanced collapse (SLAC wrist) (Fig. 3.30).

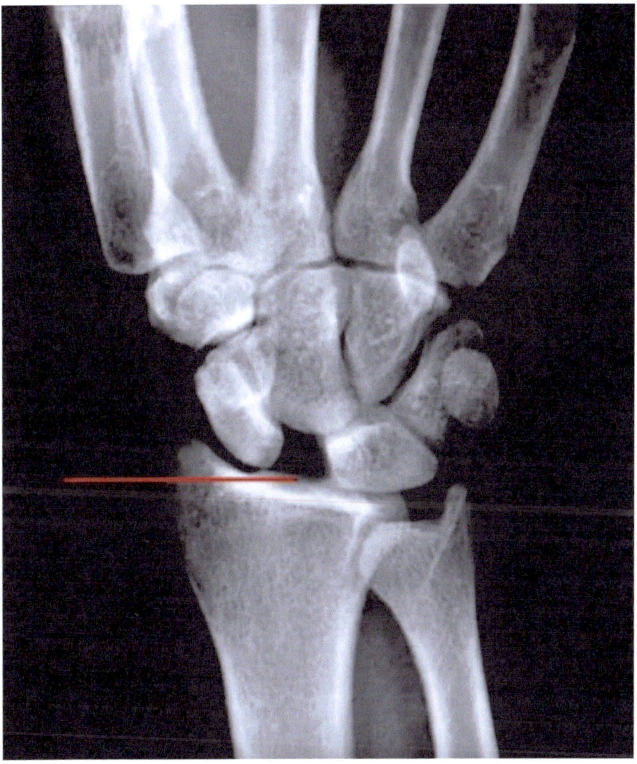

Fig. 3.29 Scapholunate gap

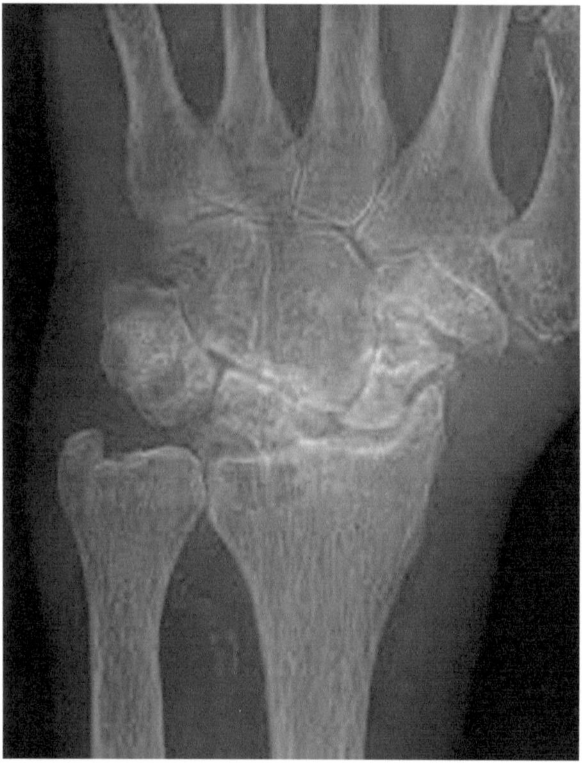

Fig. 3.30 SLAC wrist

3.7.1 Watson's Test

- Place a thumb over the tubercle of the scaphoid anteriorly (Fig. 3.31).
- On ulnar deviation and slight extension, the prominence of the tubercle disappears.
- The wrist is then moved into radial deviation while continuing to apply pressure; the scaphoid is noted to be dorsally displaced.
- The pressure on the tubercle is then released and the dorsally displaced scaphoid is felt to move back into the radial fossa.

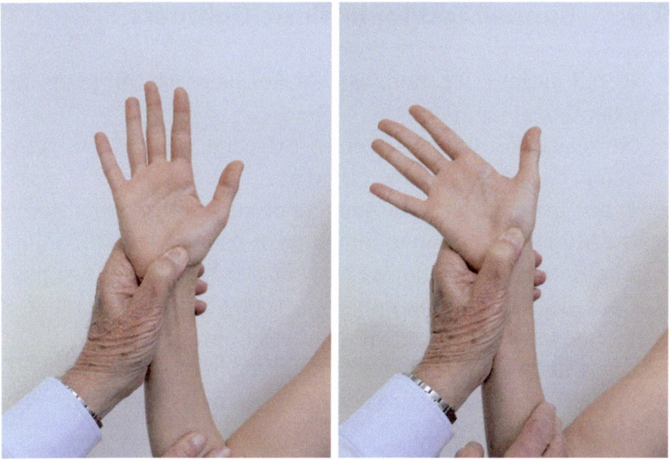

Fig. 3.31 Watson's test

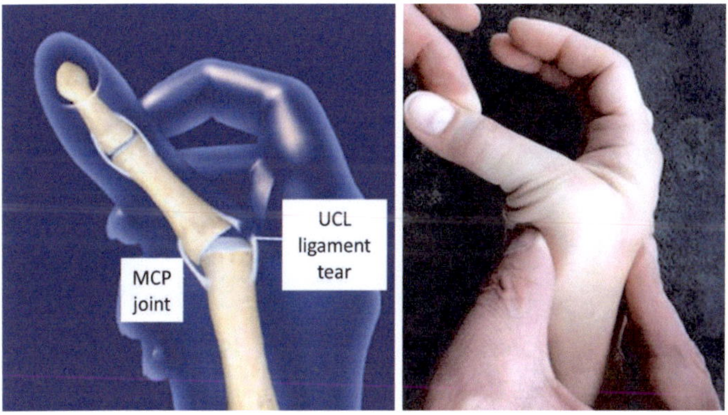

Fig. 3.32 UCL tear

3.8 Ulnar Collateral Ligament Instability of the Thumb (Gamekeeper's Thumb)

- Due to either avulsion of a piece of bone or tearing of the ligament (Fig. 3.32)

3.9 Bunnell Test for Intrinsic Tightness

- Recall intrinsic function, namely, flexion at the MP joints and extension at the IP joints.
- Normally when the MP joint is extended, there is free active and passive flexion at the PIP joint.
- When there is intrinsic tightness or contracture, extension at the MP joint will lead to limitation of flexion at the PIP joint.
- The Bunnell test is carried out with the MP joint in two positions, flexion and extension, while testing for PIP joint range of motion in both of these MP joint positions.
- There are four possibilities as indicated in the Table below.
- Go over the four situations described, as once grasped, the concepts are very satisfying!

MP joint in extension	MP joint in flexion	Diagnosis
Normal PIP flexion	Normal PIP flexion	Normal
Limited PIP flexion	Normal PIP flexion	Intrinsic tightness
Normal PIP flexion	Limited PIP flexion	Extrinsic (extensor) tightness
Limited PIP flexion	Limited PIP flexion	PIP joint pathology

4 Axillary Nerve Lesion with Deltoid Paralysis

How is it possible to obtain near normal shoulder function after permanent loss of axillary nerve function with complete deltoid atrophy?

A review of the literature written up in the journal *Military Medicine* (March 2016) [1] presented a patient with a closed axillary nerve injury. The case report describes a 43-year-old male who was involved in a motor vehicle accident at the age of 18 sustaining a dislocation of his left shoulder and an axillary nerve lesion which proved to be complete. Four years after the injury, he enlisted in the US Army with no limitation of function in his left shoulder; he was able to perform 65 push up repetitions in 2 minutes (with 100 being the highest score obtainable). There was no pain or dysfunction and on examination; there was a full range of shoulder movement with absent sensation in the axillary nerve distribution; and X-rays and MRI were normal apart from showing complete atrophy of the deltoid. Electromyographic (EMG) studies confirmed complete deltoid paralysis.

The authors raised the issue of the role of the supraspinatus in the deltoid-deficient shoulder. They did not however suggest how this remarkable return of shoulder function had occurred. They also reviewed the literature and, leaving out those cases treated surgically and those without a proper follow-up, they reported 43 cases of loss of deltoid function following axillary

R. Pillemer, *Physical Signs in Orthopedic and Neurologic Disorders*, https://doi.org/10.1007/978-3-031-99529-3_4

nerve lesion injury. Of these, 17 had a partial or complete recovery, leaving 26 cases of permanent paralysis. A total of 15 cases with complete permanent paralysis of the deltoid regained full active range of movement with good shoulder function. One case returned to professional football and another to collegiate football. Once again, however, there is no suggestion of a possible mechanism for the excellent return of shoulder function in these cases.

One of the leading textbooks on the shoulder is acknowledged to be Rockwood & Matsen's *The Shoulder* [2]. In the third edition, the authors note that:

> Young patients may be able to compensate for complete deltoid paralysis and can often perform activities of daily living with only partial disability.

Once again, no explanation is given but they do note that:

> The shoulder can easily maintain a full range of motion with an intact rotator cuff.

These sentences are repeated in the latest edition of the book.

They do not make it clear whether the intact rotator cuff is necessary for there to be a full range of movement or whether they feel that the intact cuff accounts for the recovery of a full range of movement, which seems highly unlikely.

Figure 4.1 shows the typical appearance of a patient with an axillary nerve lesion and deltoid wasting and prominence of the greater tuberosity of the humerus.

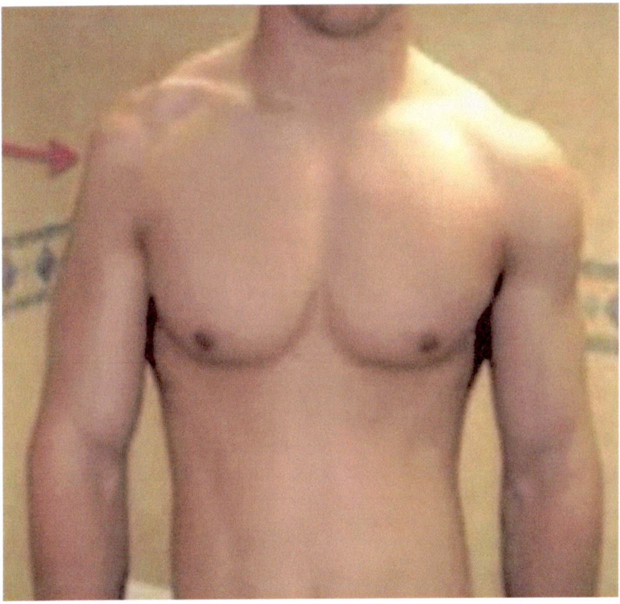

Fig. 4.1 Patient with axillary nerve lesion showing deltoid wasting and prominence of the greater tuberosity of the humerus

4.1 Anatomy of the Axillary Nerve

Reviewing the anatomy, the axillary nerve is a branch of the posterior cord of the brachial plexus which passes backwards through the quadrilateral space together with the posterior humeral circumflex artery as shown in Fig. 4.2. The space is bounded superiorly by the teres minor muscle, inferiorly by the teres major, medially by the long head of triceps, and laterally by the humeral shaft.

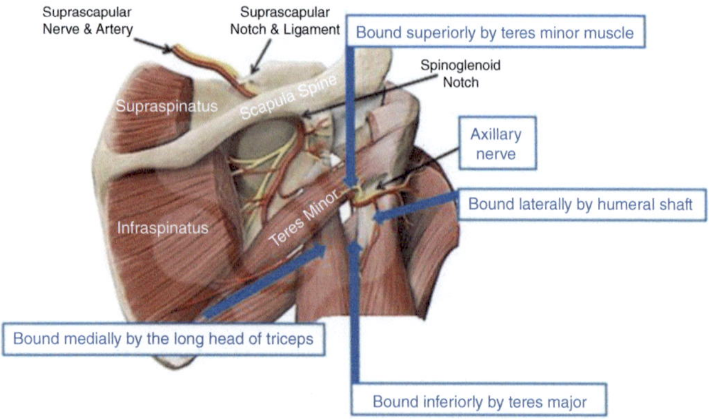

Fig. 4.2 Anatomy of the shoulder showing the axillary nerve and anatomy that bounds the quadrilateral space. (Adapted from shoulderdoc.co.uk)

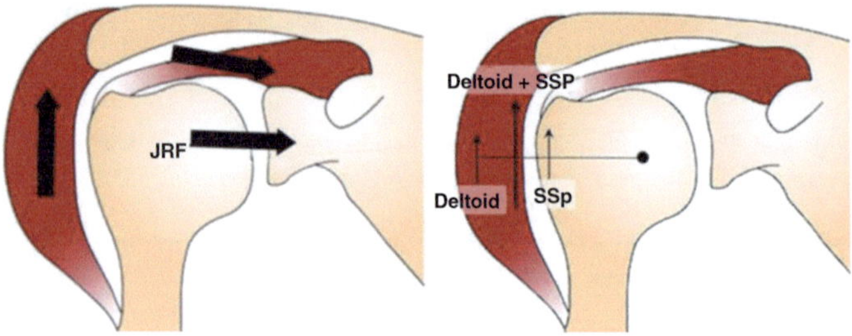

Fig. 4.3 Mechanism of abduction of the normal shoulder

4.2 Mechanism of Abduction

Abduction in the normal shoulder involves contraction of both the deltoid and supraspinatus such that, as the arm is abducted, the resultant force is directed towards the glenoid. The action of supraspinatus compresses the head of the humerus against the glenoid and maintains stability of the joint while the arm is abducted by the deltoid muscle (Fig. 4.3).

4.3 Explanation

So, how can this phenomenon of full range of shoulder movement, with particularly good power, in the presence of complete axillary nerve damage with deltoid wasting, be explained?

The suggestion is made that deltoid function is taken over by the long head of biceps. Experienced shoulder surgeons occasionally note at operation a biceps tendon that is three to four times its normal size.

This hypothesis can be supported in a patient with deltoid paralysis with a reasonable, but not full, return of function using a three-step test (Fig. 4.4):

- With his elbow flexed to 90° and with his forearm in full supination (which shortens the biceps and weakens its efficiency), he was only able to abduct to 90° (Fig. 4.4a).
- With his elbow flexed and his arm pronated (which slightly lengthens the biceps and increases its efficiency), and he was then able to abduct to 115° (Fig. 4.4b).
- With his elbow extended (further increasing efficiency), the patient was able abduct his shoulder to 135° (Fig. 4.4c).

And these findings could be readily reproduced.

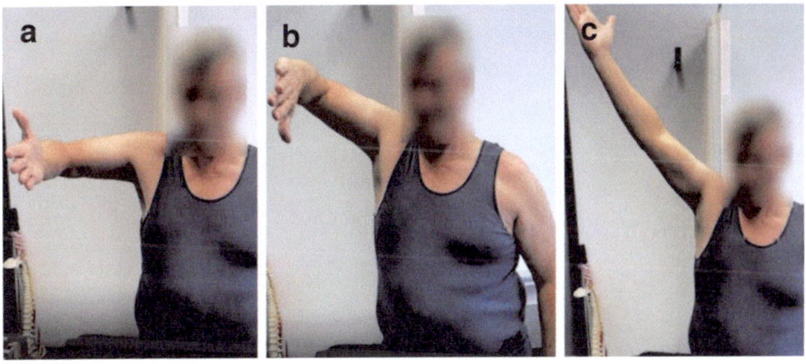

Fig. 4.4 (**a**) Abduction to 90° with forearm in full supination. (**b**) Abduction to 115° with forearm in pronation. (**c**) Abduction to 135° with elbow extended

These findings strongly suggest that the long head of biceps can compensate for the absent deltoid and that this explains the excellent function that can occur in cases of permanent deltoid paralysis [3].

(Note that early repair of axillary nerve lesions may give very satisfactory results. Nerve repair is not indicated in chronic lesions.)

References

1. Galvin JW, Eichinger JK. Outcomes following closed axillary nerve injury: a case report and review of the literature. Mil Med. 2016;181(3):e291–7.
2. Rockwood CA, Matsen FA, Wirth M, Lippitt SB, Fehringer EV, Sperling JW. Rockwood & Matsen's 'The shoulder'. 3rd ed. Philadelphia: Elsevier; 2016.
3. Pillemer R. Axillary nerve lesions with deltoid paralysis. Mega J Case Rep. 2023;6(12):2001–5.

5 Lesions of the Posterior Branch of the Axillary Nerve

Axillary nerve lesions are usually caused by trauma, such as dislocations of the shoulder or fractures of the proximal humerus. Most of these lesions are due to neuropraxia and recover within a year. Apart from these situations, the literature suggests that axillary nerve lesions are uncommon.

However, lesions of the posterior branch of the axillary nerve are quite common, and the diagnosis is simply being missed. The key to making the diagnosis is the finding of diminished sensation over the deltoid muscle in the area supplied by the axillary nerve (Fig. 5.1).

This condition was first documented in an article published in July 2023 [1] and put forward as a new syndrome.

Lesions of the posterior branch of the axillary nerve will be discussed under the following headings:

- Anatomy
- Mechanism of injury
- Clinical presentation
- Diagnosis
- Clinical significance

R. Pillemer, *Physical Signs in Orthopedic and Neurologic Disorders*,
https://doi.org/10.1007/978-3-031-99529-3_5

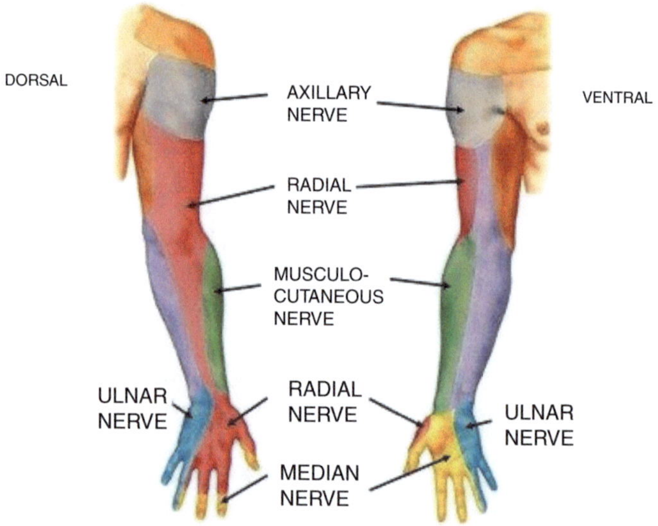

Fig. 5.1 Sensory supply of the axillary nerve

5.1 Anatomy

- The axillary nerve is one of the two terminal branches of the posterior cord of the brachial plexus (C5 and C6) the other branch being the radial nerve (Fig. 5.2).
- The nerve passes backwards through the quadrilateral space together with the posterior humeral circumflex artery. The space is bounded superiorly by the teres minor muscle, inferiorly by teres major, medially by the long head of triceps, and laterally by the humeral shaft (Fig. 5.3).
- Distal to subscapularis the nerve divides into anterior and posterior branches. The anterior branch contains all of the fibres that supply the anterior and lateral deltoid. *The posterior branch contains all the fibres to the posterior deltoid as well as all the sensory fibres.*
- Note that lesions of the of the axillary nerve itself, if severe enough, will result in wasting of the whole of the deltoid muscle, whereas lesions of the posterior branch of the nerve, *only involve the posterior deltoid* (Fig. 5.4a).

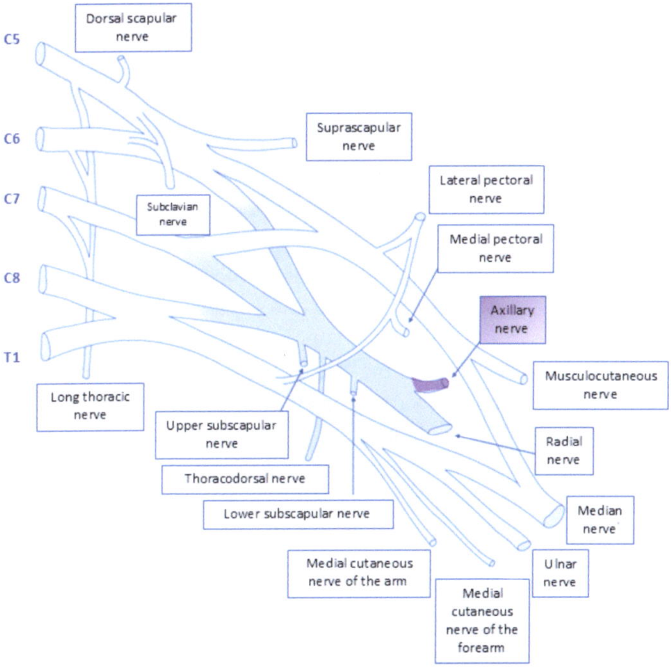

Fig. 5.2 Terminal branch of the brachial plexus

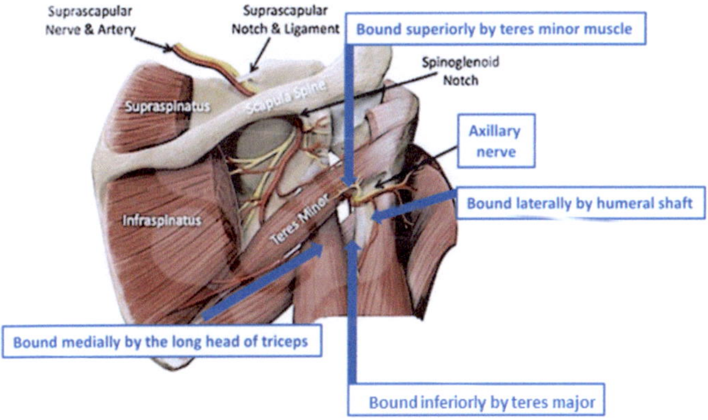

Fig. 5.3 Anatomy of the axillary nerve and the quadrilateral space

5.2 Mechanism of Injury

- The majority of cases occur as a result of a traction injury to the arm.

5.3 Clinical Presentation

- The key finding is sensory loss over the lateral aspect of the upper arm overlying the deltoid and is present in all cases.
- As the posterior branch only supplies the posterior deltoid, this is the only muscle wasting that occurs. It is not present in all cases. Compare the wasting in (Fig. 5.4a) with the unaffected right shoulder (Fig. 5.4b).
- Very commonly, there is an area of localised tenderness posteriorly over the course of the axillary nerve in relation to the lower part of the glenohumeral joint.

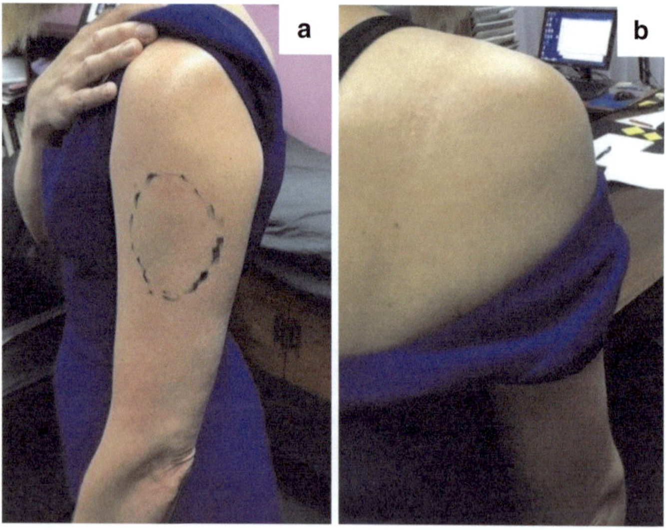

Fig. 5.4 (**a**) Wasting of the posterior deltoid (left shoulder) and (**b**) normal right shoulder

- Another example of posterior deltoid wasting on the right side (Fig. 5.5a) compared to the normal left shoulder (Fig. 5.5b), and the posterior view showing the slight concavity on the right compared to the slight convexity on the left (Fig. 5.5c).
- It is most important to stress that if careful sensory testing is not carried out in all cases of 'non-specific' post-traumatic shoulder pain, the diagnosis will be missed.

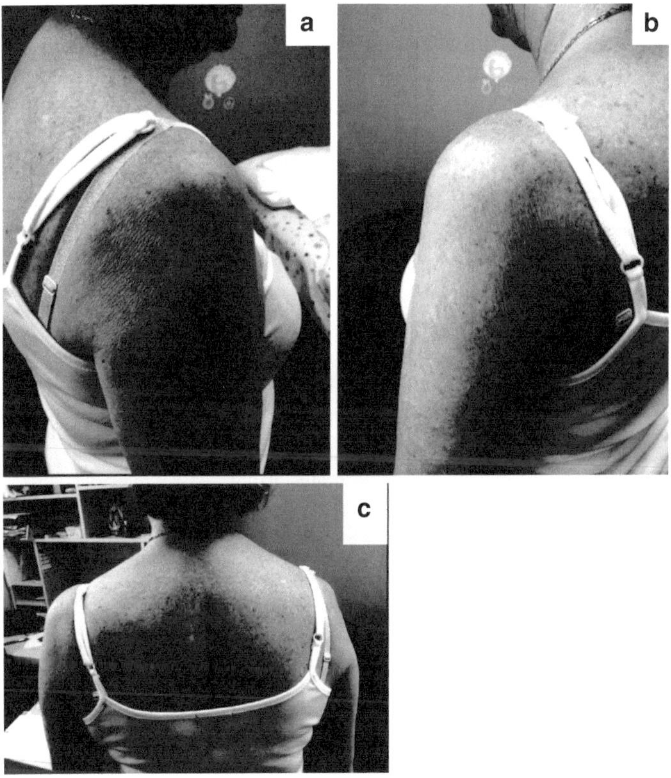

Fig. 5.5 (**a**) Right affected side; (**b**) left unaffected side; (**c**) comparison posterior view

5.4 Diagnosis

- Diminished sensation over the deltoid.
- Wasting of the posterior deltoid—pathognomonic.
- Tenderness to palpation over the axially nerve in relation to the inferior glenohumeral joint.

5.5 Clinical Significance

- The importance of this condition is that its 'non-diagnosis' may explain why ill-advised but frequently undertaken sub-acromial decompression for isolated so-called sub-deltoid bursitis reported on ultrasound or MRI fails to relieve associated symptoms.
- It is hoped that the correct diagnosis would save many patients from unnecessary subacromial surgery.

If you do not think of it, you will not look for it. If you do not look for it, you will never find it.

Reference

1. Pillemer R. Lesions of the posterior branch of the axillary nerve: common, but not previously described: a new syndrome? MEGA J Case Rep. 9 July 2023 [available online here: megajournalsofcasereports.com/wp-content/uploads/2023/07/MJCR-6-2117.pdf]

6 Supraclavicular Nerve Lesions

Lesions of the anterior branch of the supraclavicular nerve (SCN) are frequently described in relation to fractures of the clavicle, skin incisions in this region, and in relation to nerve blocks.

However, lesions of the main trunk of the SCN are said to be rare, but in fact are very common, and the diagnosis is simply being missed [1].

As with lesions of the posterior branch of the axillary nerve described in the last chapter, the key to making the diagnosis is the finding of diminished sensation over the top of the shoulder in the area supplied by the SCN (Fig. 6.1).

Lesions of the supraclavicular nerve will be discussed under the following headings:

- Anatomy
- Mechanism of injury
- Clinical presentation
- Diagnosis
- Clinical significance

R. Pillemer, *Physical Signs in Orthopedic and Neurologic Disorders*, https://doi.org/10.1007/978-3-031-99529-3_6

Fig. 6.1 Area supplied by the supraclavicular nerve

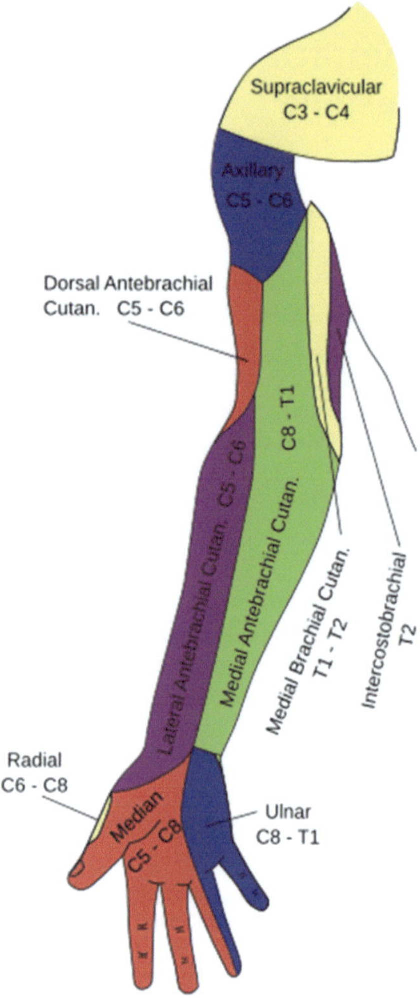

6.1 Anatomy

- The anterior rami of C3 and C4 combine to form the trunk of the SCN (Fig. 6.2) which emerges from the posterior border of sternomastoid to enter the posterior triangle of the neck (Fig. 6.3).

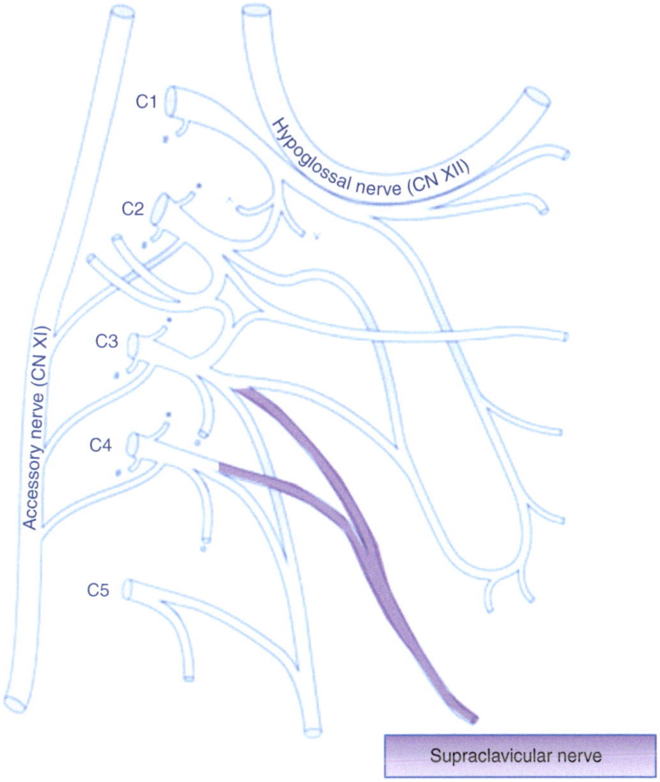

Fig. 6.2 The anterior rami of C3 and C4 combine to form the trunk of the SCN

- The nerve divides into three main branches, the anterior, lateral, and posterior (often referred to as the medial, intermediate, and lateral):
  - Anterior: supplying the anterior chest wall from the midline, over the clavicle, and as far down as the second rib.
  - Lateral: supplying the skin over the top of the shoulder, over pectoralis major and the upper deltoid.
  - Posterior: runs over trapezius supplying the skin of the posterior aspect of the shoulder.
- It is a purely sensory nerve and contributes to the innervation of the sternoclavicular joint.

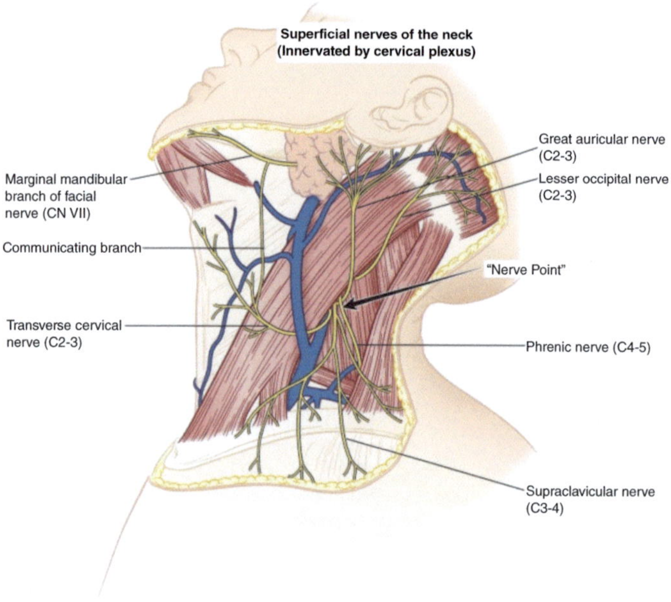

Fig. 6.3 The three main branches of the SCN

6.2 Mechanism of Injury

- Traction injuries are the most common, as well as motor vehicle accidents, and falls on to the shoulder. There was one case of a female bartender who spends much of her working time shaking cocktails with her arm in an elevated position!

6.3 Clinical Presentation

- The key finding is the diminished sensation in the distribution of the nerve, from the base of the neck, to the top of the shoulder, the anterior chest wall, upper deltoid, and the posterior shoulder (Fig. 6.4).
- Localised tenderness over the nerve as it passes behind the posterior border of the sternomastoid to enter the posterior triangle.

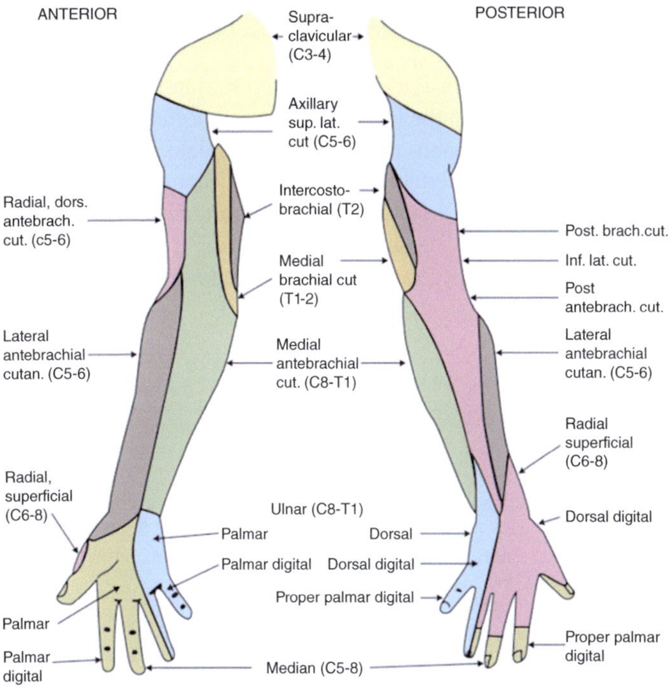

Fig. 6.4 Loss of sensation in the distribution of the supraclavicular nerve

- Percussion of the nerve in this situation commonly causes parathesias to radiate in the distribution of the nerve. Positive Tinel's sign.

6.4 Diagnosis

- Diminished sensation in the distribution of the SCN.
- Localised tenderness where the nerve enters the posterior triangle.
- Percussion causing parasthesias in the distribution of the nerve—pathognomonic.

6.5 Clinical Significance

- As in the case of lesions of the posterior branch of the axillary nerve described in the last chapter, the importance of this condition is that its 'non-diagnosis' may explain why ill-advised but frequently undertaken subacromial decompression for isolated so-called sub-deltoid bursitis reported on ultrasound or MRI fails to relieve associated symptoms.
- It is hoped that the correct diagnosis would save many patients from unnecessary subacromial surgery.

Reference

1. Pillemer R. Supraclavicular nerve lesions: a very common condition rarely diagnosed: case presentation. MEGA J Case Rep. 30 September 2023. [Available online here: megajournalsofcasereports.com/wp-content/uploads/2023/09/MJCR-69-2135.pdf

7 Scapular Winging

Scapular winging due to nerve damage is a fairly uncommon condition, and establishing an underlying cause is often difficult. The aim of this chapter is to try to simplify this process. I have used an article on scapular winging published in *Musculoskeletal Medicine* in 2008 for the basic diagram and much of the information.[1]

7.1 Types of Scapular Winging Due to Nerve Damage

There are three main types of scapular winging due to nerve damage. The most common is due to weakness or paralysis of serratus anterior. The next most common is due to paralysis of trapezius. The least common is very rare and due to involvement of the rhomboids major and minor. Importantly, all of these muscles tend to hold the scapula against the chest wall; so, damage or denervation of any of them results in winging. This is most notable with serratus anterior involvement.

[1] Martin RM, Fish DE. Scapular winging: anatomical review, diagnosis, and treatments. *Current Reviews in Musculoskeletal Medicine*. 2008;1(1):1–11. https://doi.org/10.1007/s12178-007-9000-5.

R. Pillemer, *Physical Signs in Orthopedic and Neurologic Disorders*, https://doi.org/10.1007/978-3-031-99529-3_7

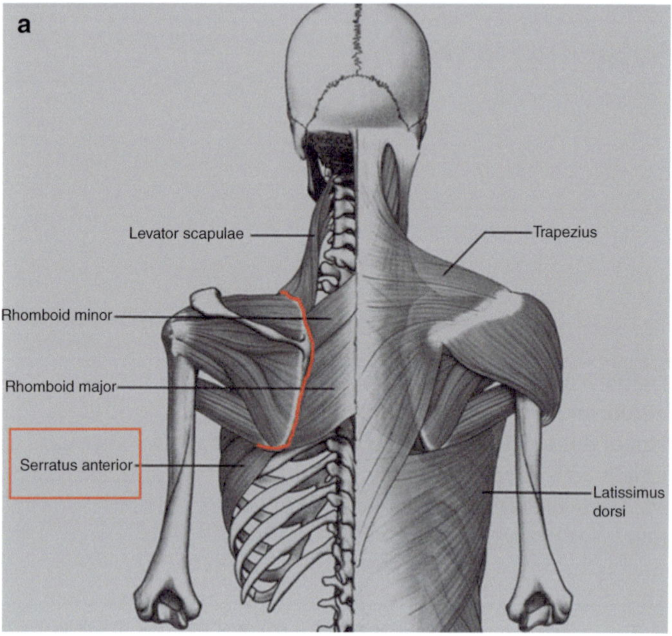

Fig. 7.1 Scapular winging may occur due to weakness or paralysis of serratus anterior

Figure 7.1 indicates that serratus anterior arises from the upper 8 ribs, lies adjacent to the side wall of the thorax, and attaches to the superior angle vertebral border and inferior angle of the scapula. When serratus anterior contracts, it pulls the scapula laterally. It is therefore easy to visualise that when the muscle is paralysed the scapula moves medially and is associated with the appearance of 'winging'.

Figure 7.2 indicates that trapezius arises in the midline from the base of the skull down to the lower thorax. It attaches to the spinous processes and supraspinous ligaments. The muscle inserts into the spine of the scapula the medial border of the acromion and also into the lateral third of the clavicle. Once again, it is easy to visualise that when the trapezius contracts the scapula is pulled medially and when it is paralysed the scapula moves laterally giving the appearance of 'winging'.

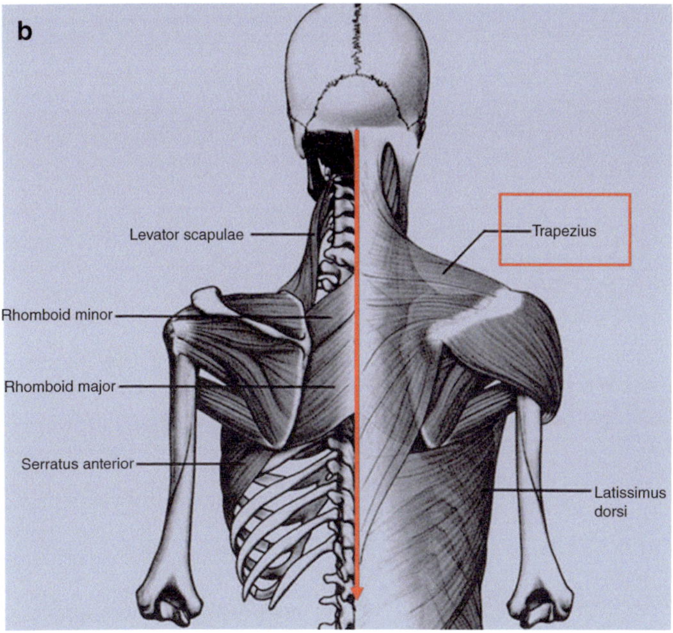

Fig. 7.2 Scapular winging may occur due to weakness or paralysis of the trapezius

Figure 7.3 indicates that the rhomboids major and minor arise from the vertebral spines and intervening spinous ligaments from C7 to T5 deep to trapezius, and insert into the medial border of the scapula. As with the trapezius, when the rhomboids contract the scapula is pulled medially and when paralysed the scapula moves laterally, again giving the appearance of 'winging'.

Note that the major difference is that in serratus anterior paralysis, the scapula moves medially, while paralysis of trapezius and the rhomboids result in the scapula moving laterally. As noted above, serratus anterior paralysis results in medial displacement and winging, whereas with trapezius and rhomboid paralysis one will get lateral displacement and winging.

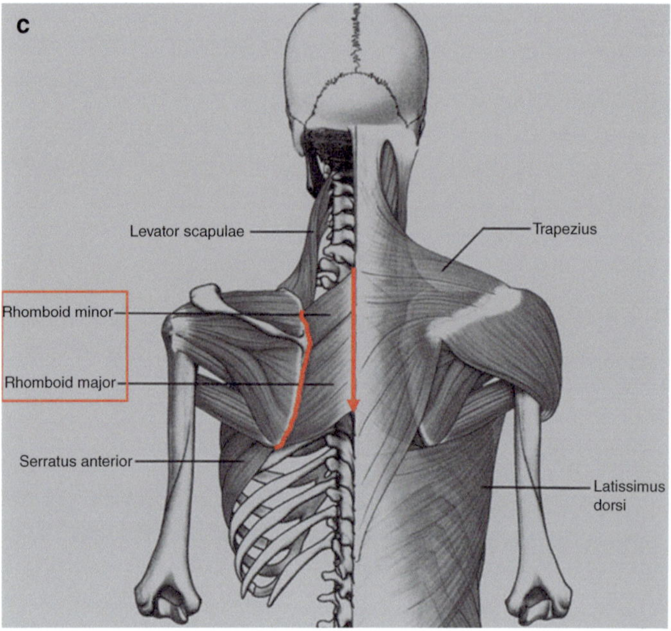

Fig. 7.3 Scapular winging may occur due to weakness or paralysis of the rhomboids. (Adapted from Martin and Fish (2008), *Musculoskeletal Medicine*)

7.1.1 Serratus Anterior Paralysis

Serratus anterior contraction not only pulls the scapula laterally but also tends to pull it downwards. Paralysis (due to loss of long thoracic nerve function) therefore also results in superior displacement of the scapula. In addition, the muscle shifts the inferior angle of the scapula more laterally assisting scapula rotation and therefore with paralysis the inferior angle displaces more medially than the superior angle.

The arrow in Fig. 7.4 demonstrates the combined effect of serratus paralysis with medial displacement, superior displacement, and medial rotation of the inferior angle.

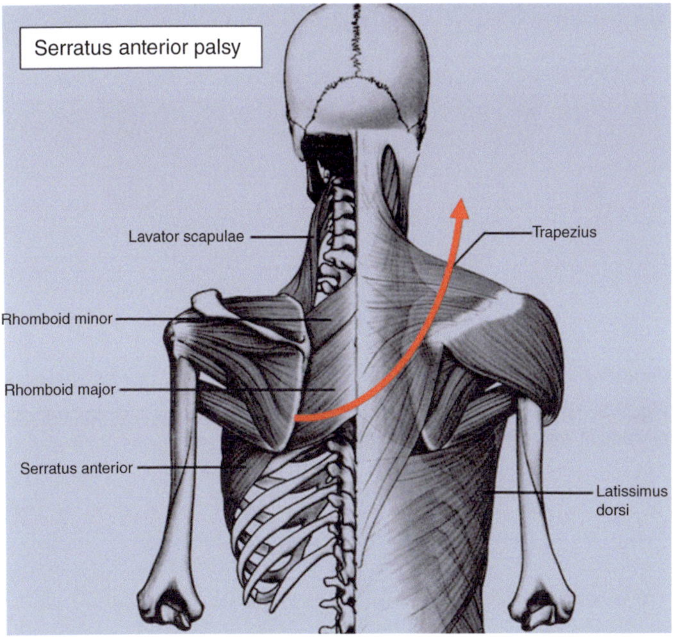

Fig. 7.4 Serratus anterior palsy with medial displacement, superior displacement, and medial rotation of the inferior angle

This is well shown in Fig. 7.5 with winging of the scapula which is displaced medially, superiorly, and with medial rotation of the inferior angle.

7.1.2 Trapezius Paralysis

The effects of trapezius paralysis (due to loss of spinal accessory nerve function) are shown in Fig. 7.6. Trapezius paralysis allows scapular winging to occur with lateral displacement. With trapezius contraction, the right scapula rotates in an anti-clockwise direction pulling the superior angle of the scapula more medially. Therefore, with paralysis of the trapezius, the superior angle will rotate more laterally.

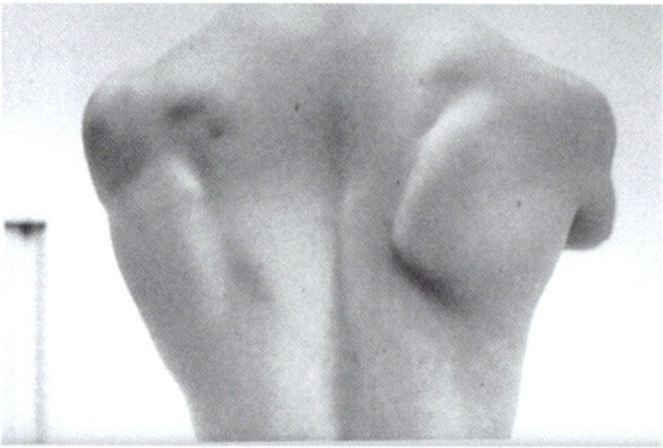

Fig. 7.5 Example of winging of the scapula with medial and superior displacement and medial rotation of the inferior angle

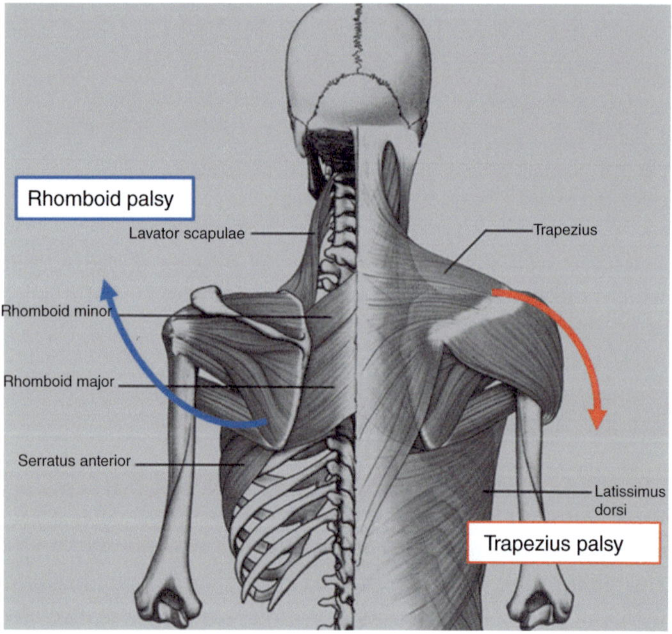

Fig. 7.6 Trapezius palsy allows scapular winging to occur with lateral displacement

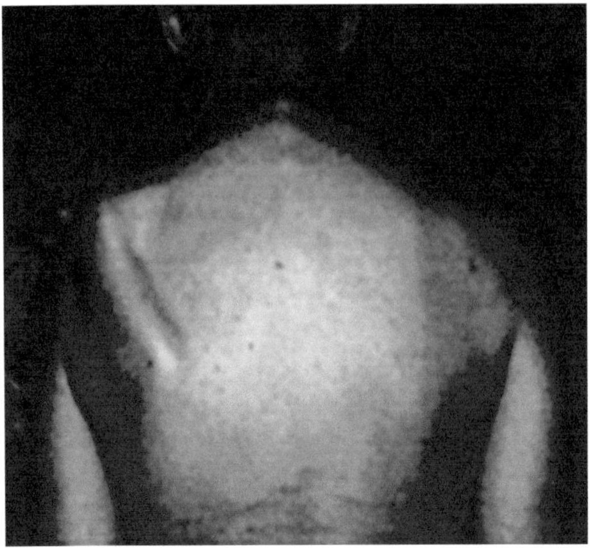

Fig. 7.7 Trapezius paralysis with winging of the scapula with lateral displacement and lateral rotation of the superior angle

A photograph is shown in Fig. 7.7 of a case of trapezius paralysis with winging of the scapula as well as lateral displacement and lateral rotation of the superior angle.

7.1.3 Rhomboid Paralysis

With rhomboid paralysis (due to loss of function of the nerves to the rhomboids), there will also be lateral displacement. Normally, contraction of the rhomboids will rotate the inferior angle medially. With paralysis, the inferior angle will rotate more laterally, and there will also be superior displacement of the scapula (Fig. 7.6).

Figure 7.8 depicts the effect of rhomboid paralysis with lateral displacement of the scapula as well as elevation and lateral rotation of the inferior angle.

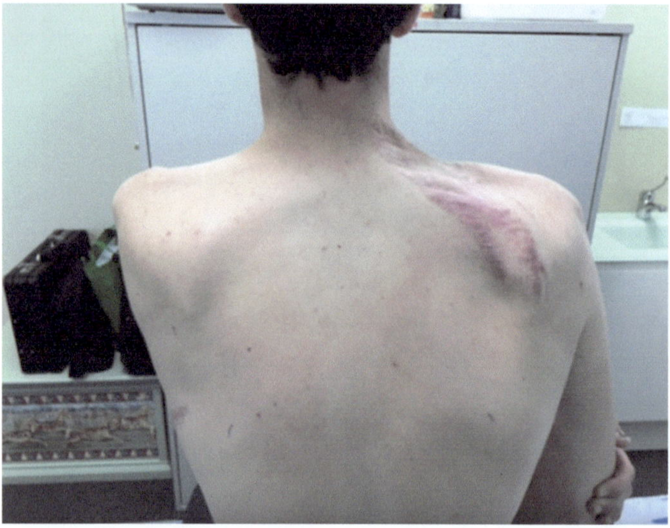

Fig. 7.8 Rhomboid paralysis with lateral displacement of the scapula as well as lateral rotation of the inferior angle

7.2 Common Tests

Common tests used to highlight winging in each of the three types of palsy noted above are shown in Fig. 7.9.

To reveal serratus anterior palsy, the patient should face a wall and take their full weight on both hands and then do a press up against the wall (Fig. 7.9a). Alternatively, the patient can press their palms firmly together at the level of the lower sternum (Fig. 7.9b).

To diagnose trapezius winging, the best method is to stand behind the patient with their elbows flexed and to resist external rotation by restraining the patient's forearms (Fig. 7.9c).

To diagnose rhomboid winging, resist extension of the shoulder as shown in (Fig. 7.9d).

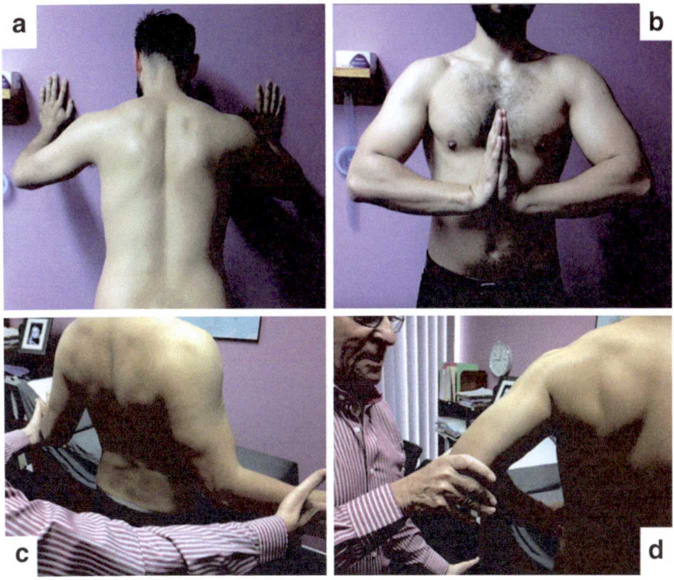

Fig. 7.9 Clockwise from top left: (**a**) serratus anterior palsy test leaning against wall, (**b**) pressing palms firmly together, (**c**) resisting extension of shoulder, (**d**) resisting external rotation

7.2.1 Summary

Figure 7.10 summarises the three types of palsy and the methods for testing each. The nerve supply for each of the three muscles is also included for completeness.

Whenever a patient with shoulder discomfort or dysfunction is assessed, the patient must always be examined from behind with their shirt or blouse removed in order to determine if there is scapula winging. As with so many other conditions, if you do not specifically look for scapula winging you will never find it.

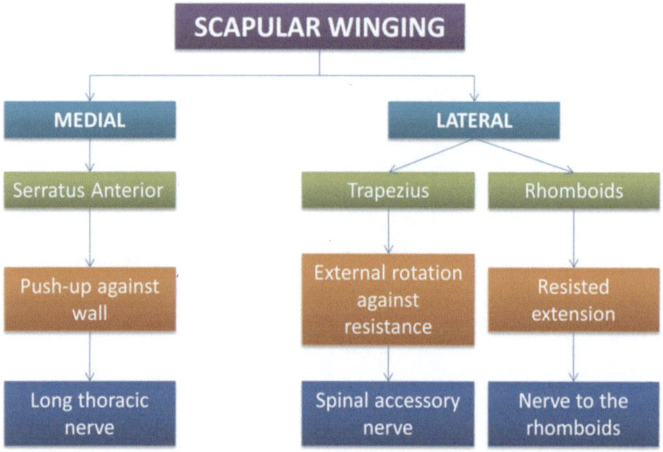

Fig. 7.10 Summary of types of scapula winging, emphasising displacement, with methods for testing and the nerve supply of the muscles

Medial Hamstring Reflex (MHR)

8

8.1 L5 Radiculopathy

Although the medial hamstring reflex (MHR) is well written up in the literature, one hardly ever sees it mentioned in medical reports. It has been established that the L5 nerve root supports the MHR, which means that we are not utilising a very useful physical sign!

The explanation for the lack of use is that it is only in the last 10 years or so that the reliability of the MHR as being supplied by the L5 nerve root has been finally established. This chapter then is to stress the importance and value of the MHR in testing for L5 radiculopathy.

I have found that the best position and method for testing the MHR is:

- With the patient supine.
- The hip slightly flexed, abducted, and externally rotated, and the knee flexed to 50–60°.
- The examiner's index and middle fingers are placed over the medial hamstring tendons (semimembranosus and semitendinosus), a few centimetres above the knee (Fig. 8.1).
- The examiner's fingers are then struck with the patella hammer; if the reflex is present, one sees the hamstrings contract and this contraction can be felt [1].

R. Pillemer, *Physical Signs in Orthopedic and Neurologic Disorders*, https://doi.org/10.1007/978-3-031-99529-3_8

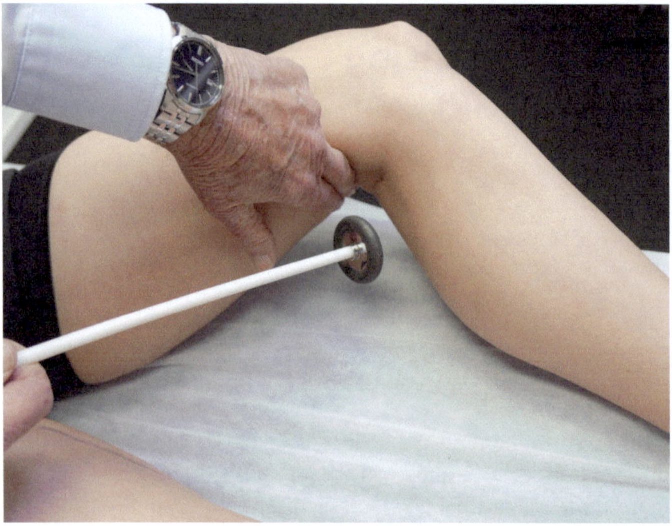

Fig. 8.1 Testing for the medial hamstring reflex

Testing for L5 radiculopathy includes the following (see Chap. 9):

- Motor: Weakness of extensor hallucis longus (EHL).
- Sensory: Diminished sensation over the lateral border of the distal leg onto the dorsum of the foot.
- Reflex: Depression/absence of MHR (always compare with the opposite side).

8.1.1 Other Less Common Signs of L5 Nerve Root Involvement

8.1.1.1 Extensor Digitorum Brevis (EDB)

Extensor digitorum brevis is supplied by the terminal branch of the deep peroneal (fibula) nerve (L5).

The muscle belly of EDB '*can be seen in most feet and felt in all*' [2], by resisted extension of the medial four toes (Fig. 8.2).

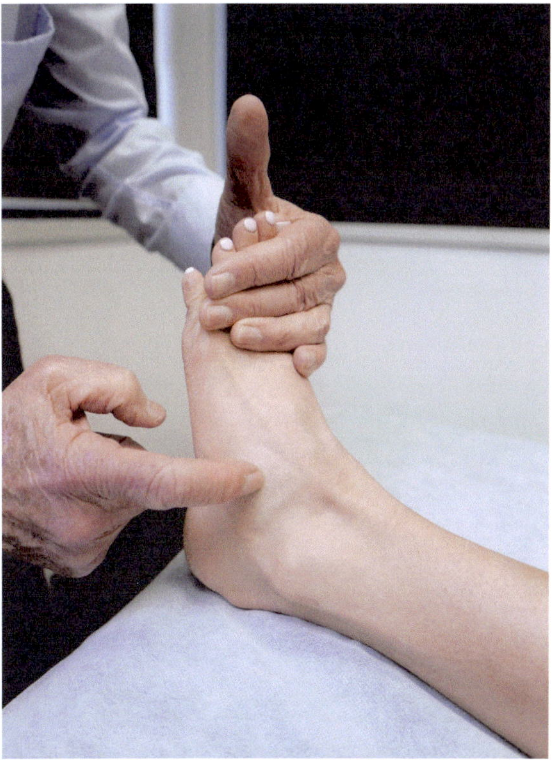

Fig. 8.2 Muscle belly of extensor digitorum brevis (EDB)

The muscle arises from the dorsal/upper surface of the distal calcaneus (Fig. 8.3), and passes obliquely across the foot to insert into the lateral aspect of extensor digitorum longus (EDL) tendons, to the second, third, and fourth toes (Fig. 8.4).

The medial part of the muscle is known as extensor hallucis brevis (EHB) which inserts into the dorsum of the base of the proximal phalanx of the big toe (Fig. 8.4).

These muscles and tendons pass deep to the tendons of extensor digitorum longus (EDL) (Fig. 8.5).

Wasting of EDB is shown in patients with L5 nerve lesions (Figs. 8.6 and 8.7).

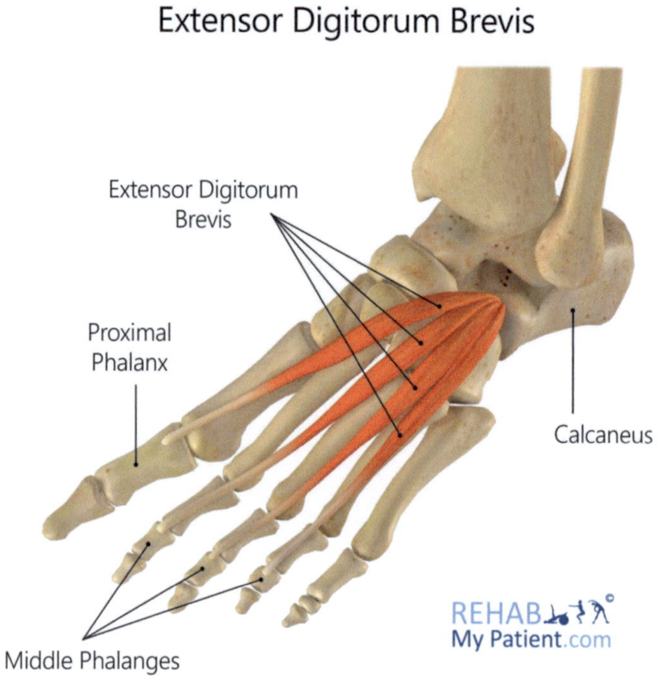

Fig. 8.3 Origin of extensor digitorum brevis (EDB)

8.1.1.2 Peroneal Reflex

Originally described by Louis Berlin [3], this reflex is subserved by the peroneal nerve (L5), and is often difficult to elicit and not always present.

The reflex can be demonstrated by tapping the examiner's fingers placed over the lateral aspect of the dorsum of the foot, with the foot in slight plantar flexion and inversion (Fig. 8.8).

A positive reflex would result in slight extension and eversion of the foot.

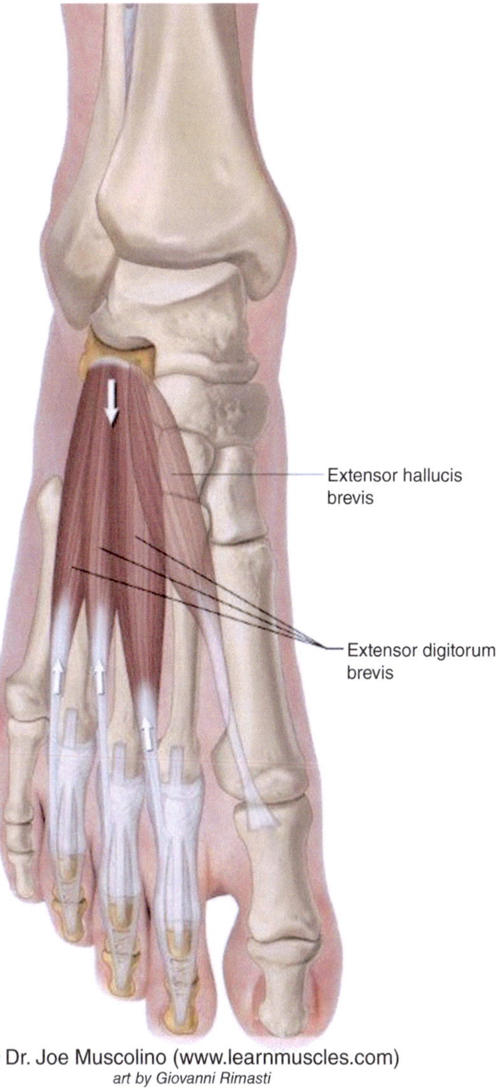

Fig. 8.4 Insertion of extensor digitorum brevis (EDB) and extensor hallucis brevis (EHB)

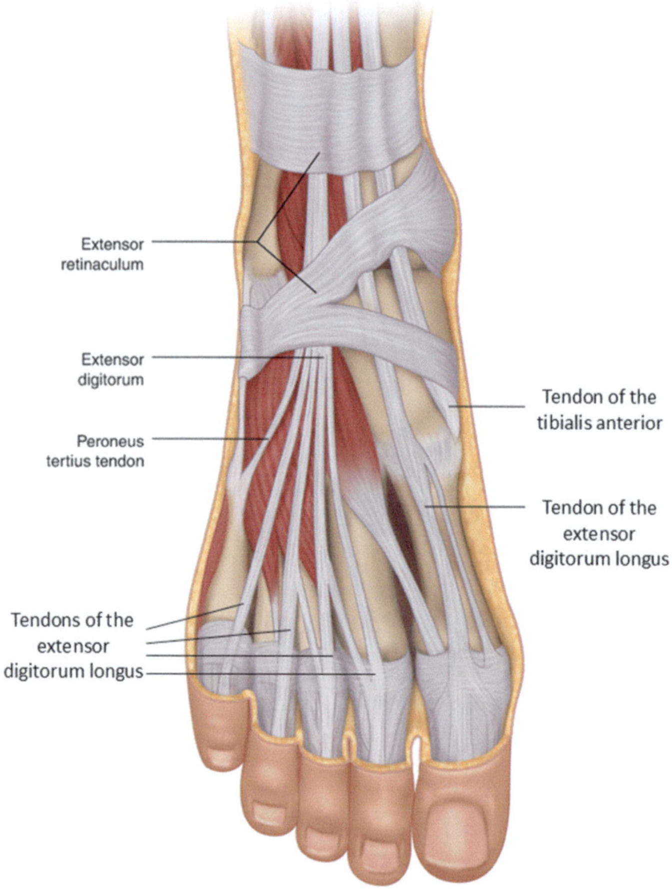

Fig. 8.5 Extensor hallucis longus (EHL) and extensor digitorum longus (EDL) insertions

8.1.1.3 How to Distinguish Between L5 Nerve Root Lesion and a Common Peroneal Nerve Lesion

It can be very difficult at times to tell the difference between an L5 nerve root lesion and a common peroneal nerve lesion (CPN) lesion. Both can present with varying degrees of foot drop and with sensory loss in a very similar distribution.

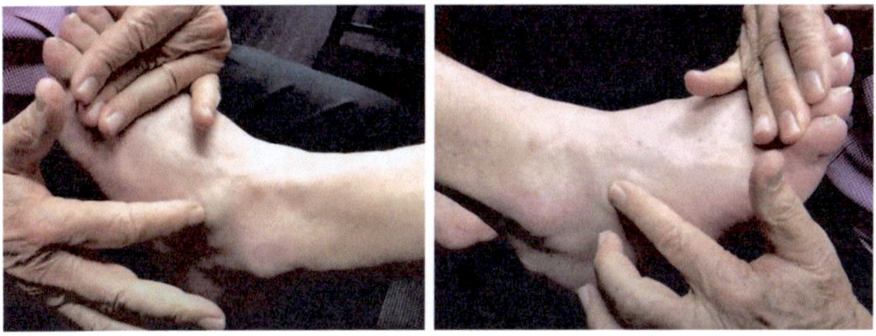

Fig. 8.6 Patient with L5 nerve root damage showing left foot with normal extensor digitorum brevis muscle and right foot with wasting/softening of the extensor brevis muscle

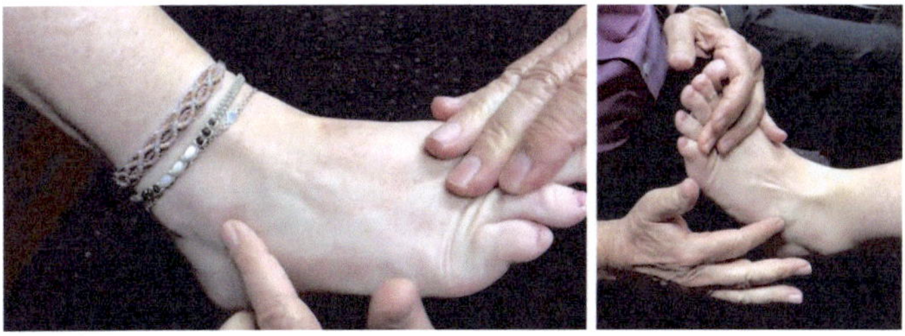

Fig. 8.7 Patient with an L5 nerve root lesion and significant wasting of the extensor digitorum brevis on the right foot, compared to normal muscle on the left foot

It is important to be aware of other causes of foot drop such as brain tumours or strokes, sciatic nerve lesions, spinal cord lesions, rupture of tibialis anterior, and various neuropathies such as diabetes.

The two commonest causes however are L5 radiculopathy and common peroneal nerve lesions.

Figure 8.9 shows the typical sensory loss in CPN lesions and the sensory loss in L5 lesions (dermatomal distribution). Remarkably similar distributions are observed. The motor loss in both conditions may produce foot drop, with weakness of ankle dorsiflexors and toe extensors, as well as weakness of ankle evertors.

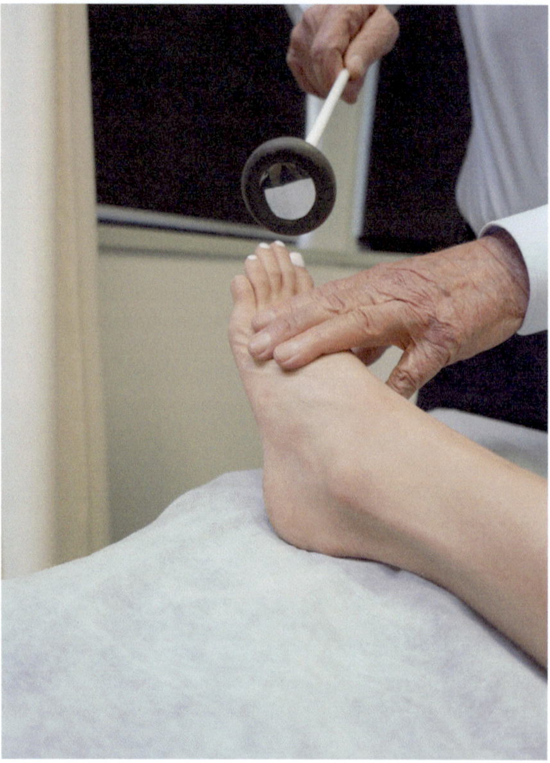

Fig. 8.8 Testing for peroneal reflex

What are the possible methods then of distinguishing between these two conditions? Five methods are suggested here:

- Limitation of straight leg raising might be present in association with L5 nerve root lesions but not with CPN lesions.
- Hip abduction: Achieved by action of gluteus medius and minimus (superior gluteal nerve) as well as piriformis. Weakness of hip abduction, with a positive Trendelenburg sign, might therefore be present in L5 nerve root lesions but not in CPN lesions.
- Medial hamstring reflex. Supplied by L5 nerve root and may therefore be depressed in L5 nerve root lesions but not in CPN lesions.

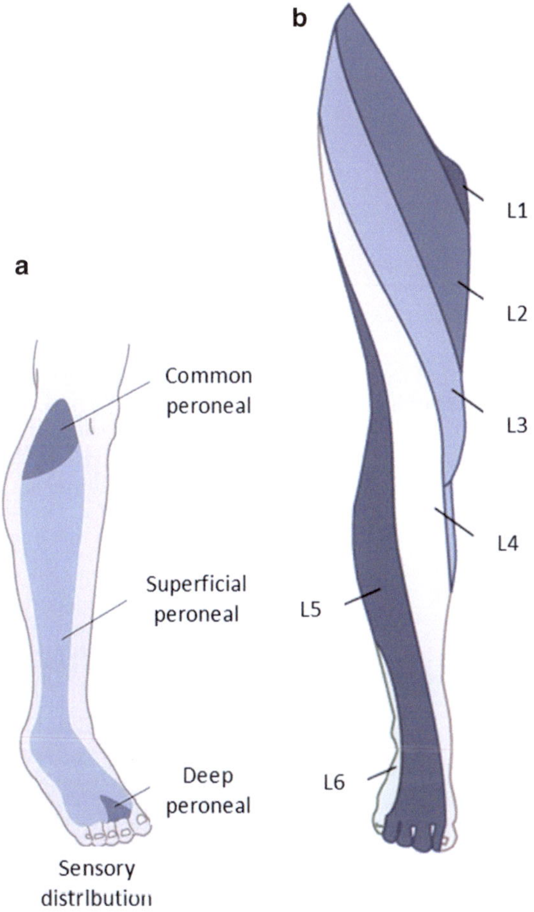

Fig. 8.9 (**a**) Sensory loss in CPN lesions. (**b**) Sensory loss in L5 nerve root lesions

- Tinel's sign. Percussion over the CPN may produce paraesthesias radiating down the leg, which will not occur in L5 nerve root lesions.
- Foot inversion. Tibialis anterior is a foot invertor and is supplied by L4 and L5. Weak inversion might therefore occur in L5 nerve root lesions but not in CPN lesions.

These differences are summarised in the table below:

	L5 nerve root	Common peroneal nerve
Straight leg raising	Restricted	Normal
Hip abduction	Weak	Normal
Medial hamstring reflex	Depressed/absent	Normal
Tinel's sign	Absent	Present
Foot inversion	Normal	Weak

References

1. Pillemer R. YouTube "In Brief" Radiculopathy Part 1. The importance of the medial hamstring reflex.
2. Sinnatamby C. Last's anatomy. 10th ed. Edinburgh: Churchill Livingstone; 1999. p. 139.
3. Berlin, L. A Peroneal Muscle Stretch Reflex. Neurology. 1971;21 (11):1177. https://doi.org/10.1212/WNL.21.11.1177

9 Lumbosacral Radiculopathy

This chapter will suggest a systematic method of examination of the common nerve roots involved in lumbosacral radiculopathy, namely, L4, L5, and S1. A careful history is undertaken in every case.

Radiculopathy: Disorder of spinal nerve roots

- Lumbosacral radiculopathy is a pain syndrome due to compression or irritation of nerve roots in the lumbosacral spine.
- It is caused by lumbar disc herniation, facet hypertrophy, spondylolisthesis, or foraminal narrowing, where the nerves exit the spinal canal.
- It is a very common presentation in musculoskeletal medicine; the majority of cases resolve spontaneously.
- However, be alert for 'red flags',[1] which require urgent attention.
- Unexplained fever, weight loss.

[1] *Red Flags*:

- Urinary retention, faecal incontinence, saddle anaesthesia which are all features of cauda equina syndrome (CES)
- Widespread/bilateral weakness, sensory or reflex loss
- Severe trauma or recent surgery
- Unexplained fever, weight loss

R. Pillemer, *Physical Signs in Orthopedic and Neurologic Disorders*, https://doi.org/10.1007/978-3-031-99529-3_9

9.1 Segmental Innervation

The spinal nerves supply three functions segmentally at each spinal level, namely, sensory, motor, and reflex functions. Tests for each of these functions will be discussed.

9.1.1 Sensory Function

- The area of skin supplied by a single spinal nerve is called a 'dermatome' (Fig. 9.1).
- While there is overlap of adjacent dermatomes, as in the upper limb, there are autonomous zones which are very specific for each nerve root (Fig. 9.2).
  - L2: anteromedial mid-thigh
  - L3: medial femoral condyle
  - L4: medial malleolus
  - L5: the skin over the third metatarsophalangeal joint on dorsum of foot
  - S1: lateral heel
  - S2: popliteal fossa, slightly medial to the midline

9.1.2 Motor Function

- The muscles supplied by a single spinal nerve is called a 'myotome.'
- The segmental innervation of muscles is described in Jack Last's textbook of anatomy; the most informative few pages I have read since starting medical school.

  In summary, Last notes the following:

- Most muscles are supplied equally from two adjacent segments of the spinal cord.
- Muscles sharing a common primary action on a joint are supplied by the same two segments.

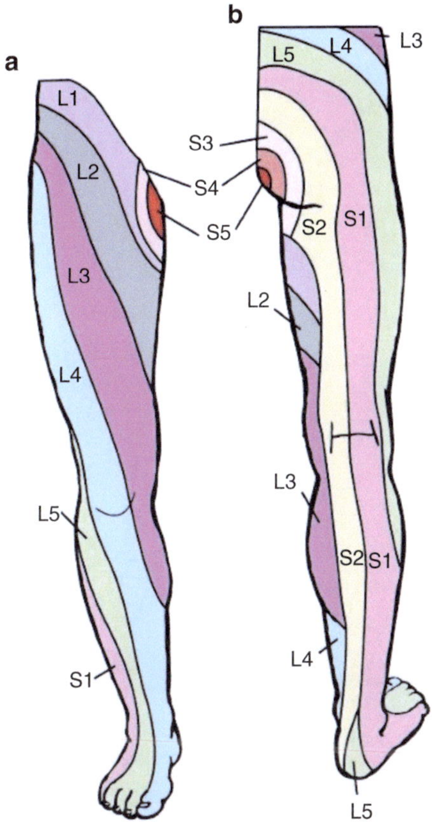

Fig. 9.1 Dermatomes of the legs (**a**. front; **b**. back)

- Their opponents, sharing the opposite action, are likewise all supplied by the same two segments which run in numerical sequence with the former.
- For a joint one segment more distal in the limb, the centre lies *en bloc* one segment lower in the cord.
- The segments mainly responsible for the various limb joint movements are summarised in Fig. 9.3.

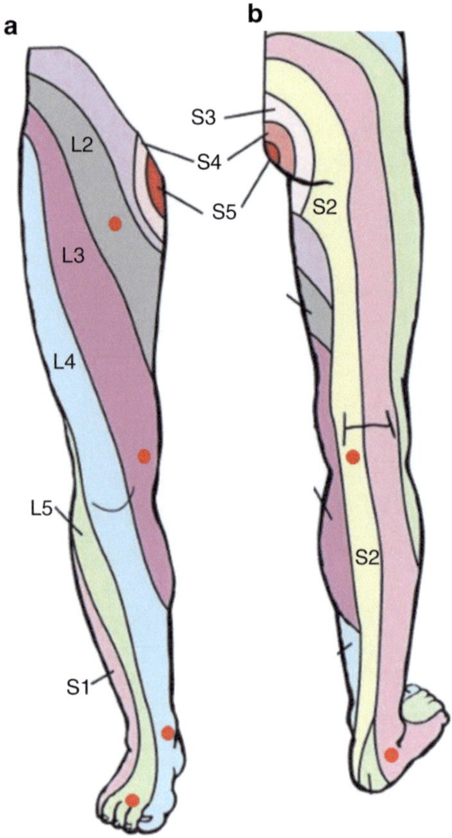

Fig. 9.2 Autonomous zones (**a**. front; **b**. back)

The above pattern enables the segmental innervation of a muscle to be determined, for example:

- Iliacus (flexes hip): L2,3
- Biceps femoris (flexes knee): L5,S1
- Soleus (plantar flexion ankle): S1,2

Last notes that the above are simply flexion-extension movements and cover all knee and ankle moving muscles.

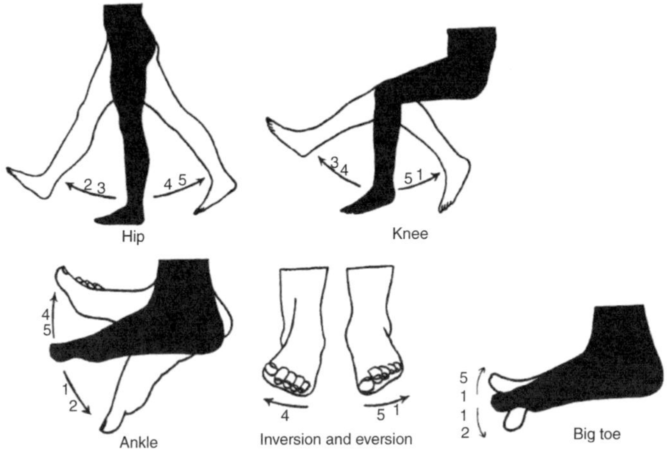

Fig. 9.3 Segmental innervation lower limb

At the hip, movements other than flexion and extension are possible, but all are innervated by the same four segments. Thus:

- Adduction or medial rotation (same as flexion): L2,3
- Abduction or lateral rotation (same as extension): L4,5
- For innervation of the foot the formula is:
  - Invert foot: L4
  - Evert foot: L5,S1

9.1.2.1 Application

- Each joint is supplied by four segments of the cord.
- As you move down a joint, you move down a segment.
- Anterior muscles contract first.
- Therefore, start the hip at L2, the knee at L3, and the ankle at L4.

Practice this a few times and you will soon know the segmental innervation of all the muscles of the lower limb!

9.1.3 Reflex Function

L4: Knee reflex
L5: Medial hamstring reflex (See Chap. 8)
S1: Ankle reflex

- If a reflex appears to be absent, retest while getting the patient to clench the teeth, forcibly trying to pull interlocked fingers apart, or squeezing the knees together (reinforcement) (Fig. 9.4).
- Hyperreflexia may indicate an upper motor neurone lesion (UMNL). Other signs include increased muscle tone, clonus, and Babinski sign.

9.1.3.1 Systematic Method of Testing for Radiculopathy

There are 6 tests for reflexes, three on each side, 6 tests for sensory dermatomes, three on each side, and 6 tests for motor power, three on each side (see Fig. 9.5). I suggest calling this the *666 method of testing for radiculopathy*.[2]

Reflexes (6 tests)

- Test for the knee, medial hamstring and ankle reflexes, on both sides.

Motor Power (6 tests)

- Test for motor power by ankle inversion, extension of the big toe, and ankle eversion, on both sides.

Sensory Testing (6 tests)

- Sensory testing over the medial malleolus, dorsum of the foot, and the lateral heel, on both sides.

---

[2]For those of you with a biblical inclination that is the sign of the 'beast' (Revelations 13:18). 666 is also the sum of all the numbers on a roulette wheel, 1–36.

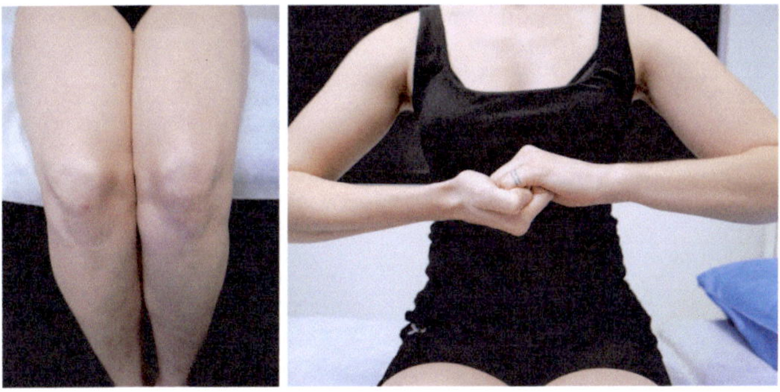

Fig. 9.4 Reinforcement

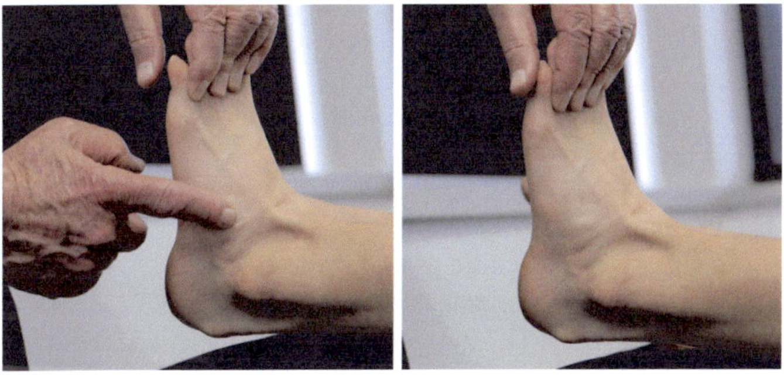

Fig. 9.5 Extensor digitorum brevis (EDB)

Table 9.1 shows the changes that might be found with involvement of the specific nerve roots (L3 has been included for completeness).

A pictorial representation of the 666 method for testing is shown in Table 9.2.

The Anatomy of the Lumbosacral Plexus (for Completeness)
As each of the nerves forming the lumbosacral plexus leave the spinal canal, they divide into anterior and posterior branches (rami), (Fig. 9.6).

The lumbar plexus is formed by the anterior rami of L1–L4, while the sacral plexus is formed by the anterior rami of S1–S4

Table 9.1 Clinical presentation of specific nerve root involvement

Nerve root	Reflex	Motor deficit	Sensory deficit
L3	Hip	Hip flexion and adduction	Medial thigh to knee
L4	Knee	Quadriceps Foot inversion	Medial leg and foot
L5	Medial hamstring	Extensor hallucis longus and extensor digitorum brevis[a] (EHL and EDB)	Anterolateral leg Dorsum of foot
S1	Ankle	Plantar flexion Eversion	Lateral foot and sole

[a]Another sign of L5 nerve root involvement that is well described but seldom referred to, is wasting of EDB. As Jack Last says this is a muscle 'whose fleshy belly can be seen in most feel and felt in all' (Fig. 9.5). It is supplied by the lateral terminal branch of the deep peroneal nerve (L5)

with a significant contribution from the lumboscral trunk (L4 and L5), (Fig. 9.6).

The lumbar plexus (Fig. 9.7):

- The plexus forms within psoas major.
- The two main motor branches are as follows:
  - Femoral nerve (L2,3,4) which supplies the quadriceps (rectus femoris and the three vasti).
  - Obturator nerve (L2,3,4) which supplies adductor longus and brevis, and the pelvic component of adductor magnus.

The main sensory branch is the saphenous nerve, a terminal branch of the femoral nerve arising in the femoral triangle. It extends all the way down the anteromedial thigh and medial lower leg, anterior to the medial malleolus, and down to the base of the big toe. Surely the longest nerve in the body! The infra-patellar branch is often damaged in anterior knee incisions. (The literature suggests that the longest nerve in the body is the sciatic nerve which forms in the sacral plexus and extends all the way down the lower extremity and into the foot. However, the sciatic nerve divides into its terminal branches in the region of the popliteal fossa, where it ceases to be the sciatic nerve) (Table 9.3).

Table 9.2 The 666 method for systematic testing for radiculopathy

Reflexes	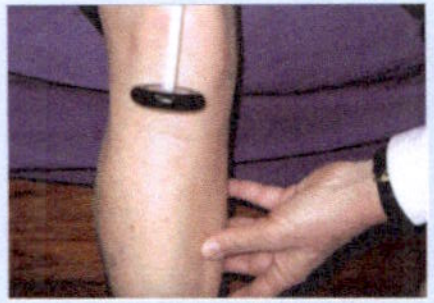		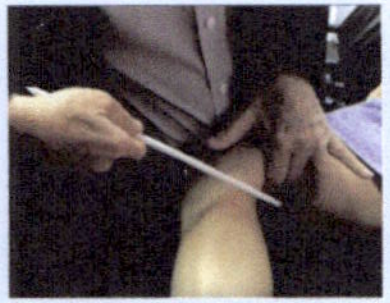		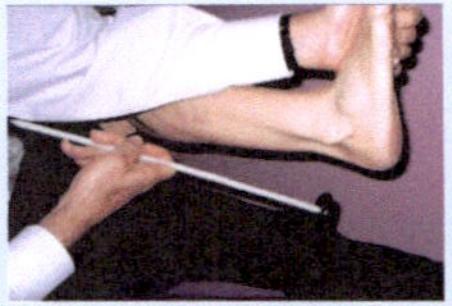	
	Knee (L4)		Medial hamstring (L5)		Ankle (S1)	
	Right side	Left side	Right side	Left side	Right side	Left side
Motor power	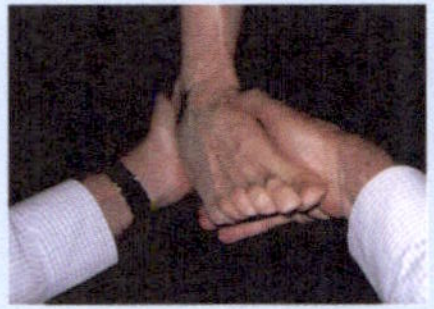		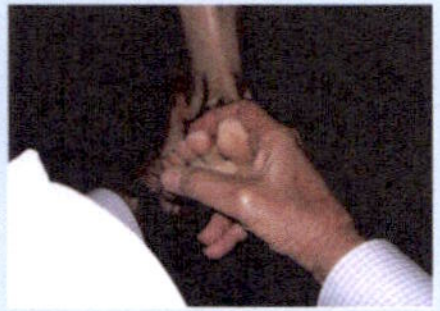		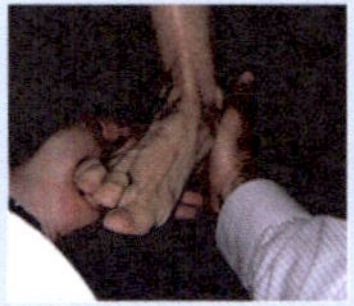	
	Inversion (L4)		Extension of the big toe (L5)		Eversion (S1)	
	Right side	Left side	Right side	Left side	Right side	Left side
Sensory testing	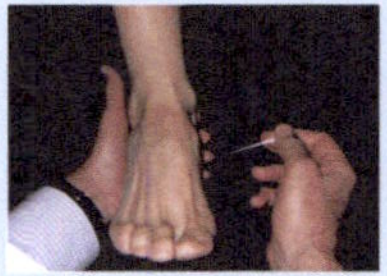		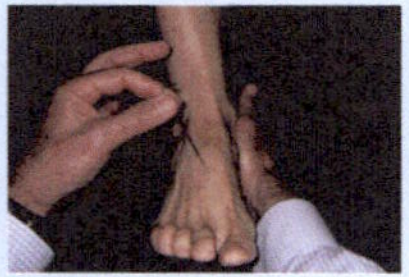		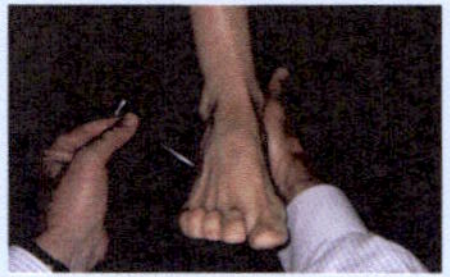	
	Inside foot (L4)		Top of foot (L5)		Outside foot (S1)	
	Right side	Left side	Right side	Left side	Right side	Left side

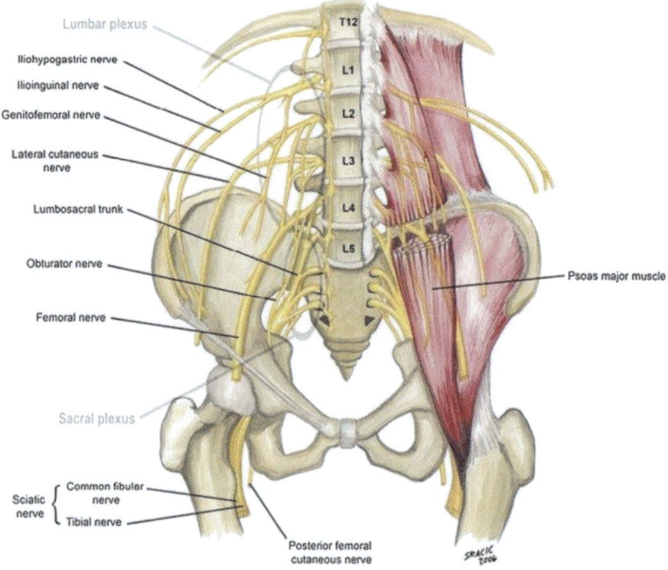

Fig. 9.6 The lumbosacral plexus

The sacral plexus (Fig. 9.8):

- Forms on the anterior aspect of piriformis muscle.
- The largest branch of the plexus is the sciatic nerve (L4,5,S1,2,3) formed by the union of its tibial and common peroneal (fibular) components.
- It innervates all the muscles of the posterior thigh (hamstrings) as well as the ischial component of the adductor magnus.
- The nerve divides into its two components in the region of the popliteal fossa, which then go on to supply all the muscles below the knee.
- Other branches of the plexus include the following:
  - The pudental nerve which supplies motor and sensory branches to the pelvic floor and perineum, including the perianal skin, the penis/clitoris, and the scrotum and vulva.
  - The superior and inferior gluteal nerves.
  - The nerve to obturator internus.

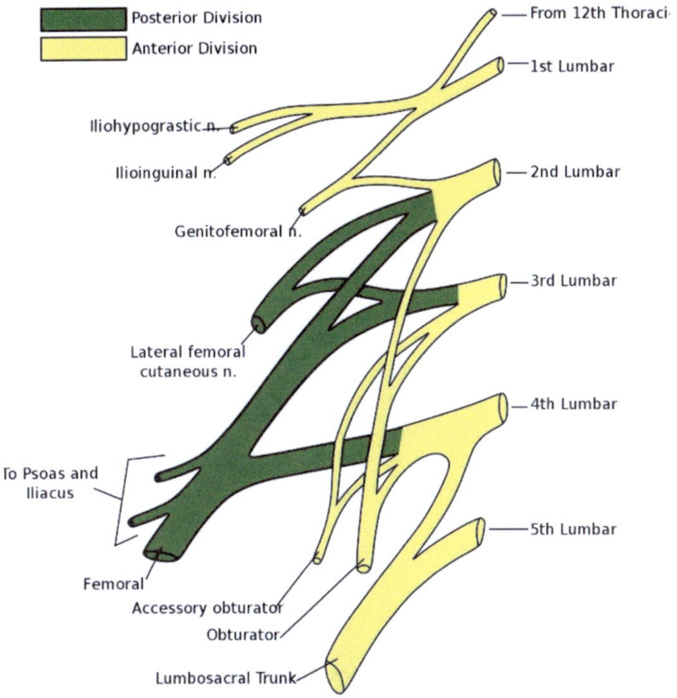

Fig. 9.7 The lumbar plexus

- The nerve to quadratus femoris.
- The perianal branch of S4.

9.1.3.2 Further Comment

I would like to stress the importance of testing the medial hamstring reflex as a sign of L5 nerve root damage. I have no doubt that if you test for this nerve root on a routine basis, you will find it an enormously useful adjunct to your testing for radiculopathy. I have also suggested a routine method for testing for the more commonly involved L4, L5, and S1 nerve roots when testing for radiculopathy. (See Roger Pillemer YouTube: L5 Radiculopathy).

I would also like to stress the importance of using a routine method of testing for the more commonly involved L4, L5, and S1 nerve roots when testing for radiculopathy.

Table 9.3 A useful mnemonic for the main branches of the lumbar plexus

Interested	In	Getting	Lunch	On	Friday
Iliohypogastric	Ilioinguinal	Genitofemoral	Lateral Femoral cutaneous	Obturator	Femoral

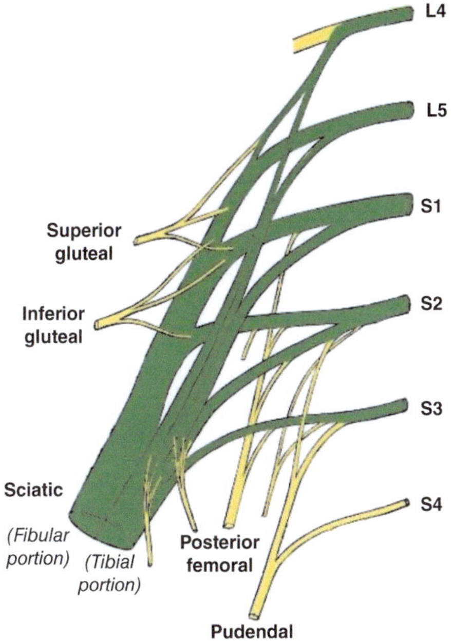

Fig. 9.8 The sacral plexus

Straight Leg Raising Test 10

10.1 An Incorrect Interpretation of Waddell's Distraction Test

The straight leg raise (SLR) test is used to detect nerve root irritation in the lumbo-sacral spine. It does this by placing tension on the sciatic nerve and then sequentially on the spinal nerve roots. Numerous studies have shown that the test has higher sensitivity than specificity, with a negative test tending to rule out radiculopathy.

The test is carried out with the patient supine and with a pillow supporting the head. The leg is then lifted passively with one of the examiner's hands supporting the heel and the foot, while the other is placed on the lower thigh keeping the knee in extension.

Always start with the unaffected leg, gradually flexing the hip, while watching the patient's face for the first signs of discomfort. A useful adjunct is dorsiflexion of the foot and ankle at this stage to see if this causes an increase in discomfort/pain (Lasegue's test).

A positive SLR test will also occur with tight hamstrings, and this is discussed below.

The SLR test plays a significant role in the medicolegal setting where it is often used to determine the veracity of the injured worker. The best-known article on non-organic signs was pub-

R. Pillemer, *Physical Signs in Orthopedic and Neurologic Disorders*, https://doi.org/10.1007/978-3-031-99529-3_10

lished by Waddell et al. in 1980.[1] Waddell received the Volvo award for clinical science for this publication and in musculoskeletal medicine we are all aware of 'Waddell's signs'. Waddell's 'Distraction test' is regarded as the gold standard in the interpretation of the SLR test.

As noted in the subtitle of this chapter, Waddell's test is being incorrectly interpreted with significant implications for the injured worker.

10.1.1 The Distraction Test

I would like to concentrate on one particular sign in Waddell's paper, namely, the distraction test. Waddell states:

> A positive physical finding is demonstrated in the routine manner. This finding is then checked when the patients attention is distracted. Any finding that is consistently present is likely to be physically based. Findings that are present only on formal examination and disappear at other times may have a non-organic component.

The example that is given under the heading 'Distraction Test' is the straight leg raising test (SLR). Waddell states:

> Straight leg raising is the most useful distraction test. Patients whose back pain has a non-organic component, show marked improvement in straight leg raising as compared to formal testing.

The reader is then referred to "Fig. 4" (Fig. 10.1) which shows the patient in a seated position with hip flexed to 90° and knee extended with the following caption: '*Straight leg raising improving with distraction, as when testing the plantar reflex in the sitting position*'.

This sign is regularly quoted in medicolegal reports as being a non-organic sign and I have never read, or heard, of this being questioned. I have, however, marked reservations about the validity of this test. I routinely find that the equivalent of straight leg

[1] Waddell G, Mc Culloch JA, Kummel E, et al. Nonorganic physical signs in low-back pain. *Spine*. 1980;5:117–25.

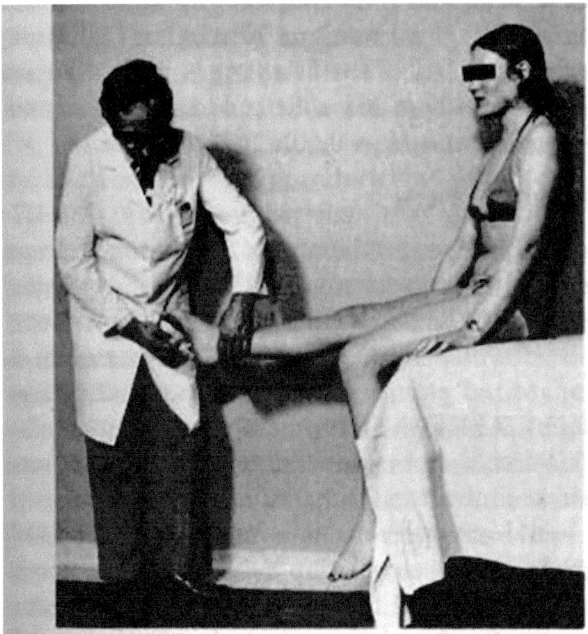

Fig 4. Straight leg raising improving with distraction, as when testing the plantar reflex in the sitting position.

Fig. 10.1 The distraction test

raising in the sitting position is greater than that demonstrated on formal examination in the supine position. This is noted to be the case even in the most genuine of patients and I cannot imagine that others have not found this as well. The discrepancy (between limited straight leg raising on formal examination in the supine position and the sitting position) even occurs in patients with signs of radiculopathy and also in those with tight hamstrings.

(Please refer to my YouTube video where four cases are shown with objective signs of radiculopathy who show an increased straight leg raising in the seated compared to the supine position.[2])

[2]Roger Pillemer YouTube: 'Testing Veracity Part 1': Video 11. https://www.youtube.com/watch?v=xZSi9Joi7xQ.

10.1.2 Case Study 1

A 30-year-old male who injured his back in 2014, with referred pain into his right foot, had had surgery in 2015. He was seen in 2019 with the following positive clinical signs (Fig. 10.2):

- Straight leg raising of 30° on the right
- Absent ankle reflex
- Decreased sensation in the S1 distribution
- Weakness of eversion of the right foot

When he sat with his legs over the side of the examining couch, a far greater range of (the equivalent of) straight leg raising was possible (Fig. 10.3).

Please note that it is most important that when sitting the patient should be instructed to hold onto the side of the examining couch to avoid extension of the spine when the leg is straightened.

10.1.3 Case Study 2

A 30-year-old security officer injured his back in 2011 unloading heavy bags of coins. He developed an S1 nerve root lesion on the left side but declined surgery. When examined in February 2017, he had the following positive clinical signs (Fig. 10.4):

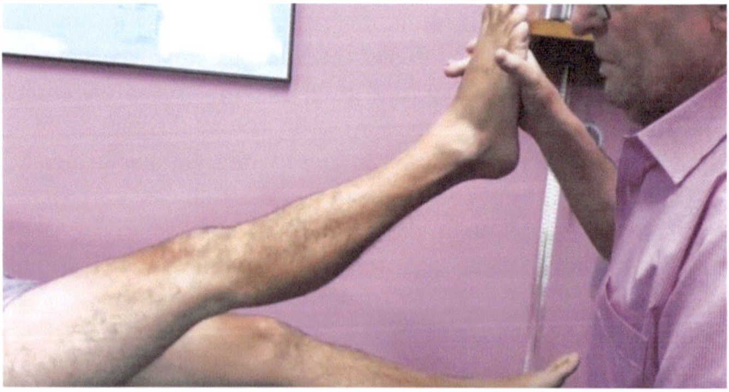

Fig. 10.2 Straight leg raising of 30° on the right in the supine position

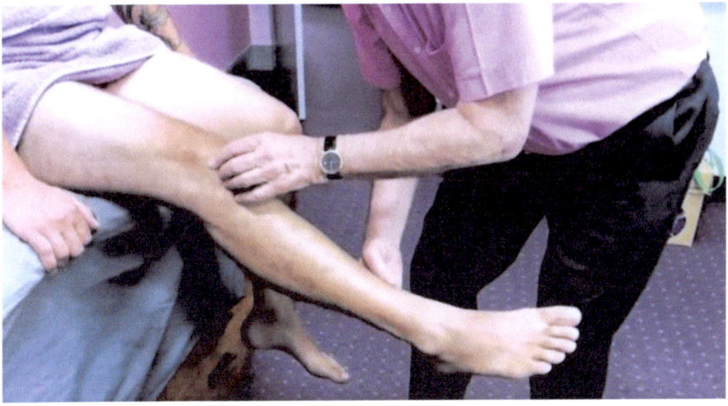

Fig. 10.3 Greater range of knee extension when seated

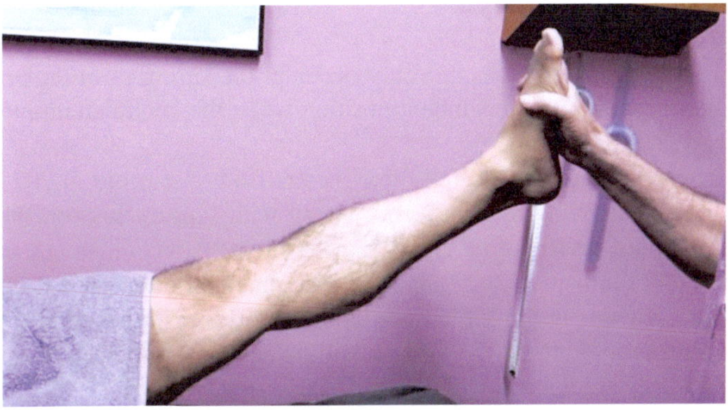

Fig. 10.4 SLR less than 30° on the left in the supine position

- SLR less than 30° on the left
- Absent ankle reflex
- Decreased sensation in the S1 distribution
- Weak eversion of the left foot

Once again note the significant restriction of SLR in the supine position compared to the greater range of SLR in the sitting position (Fig. 10.5).

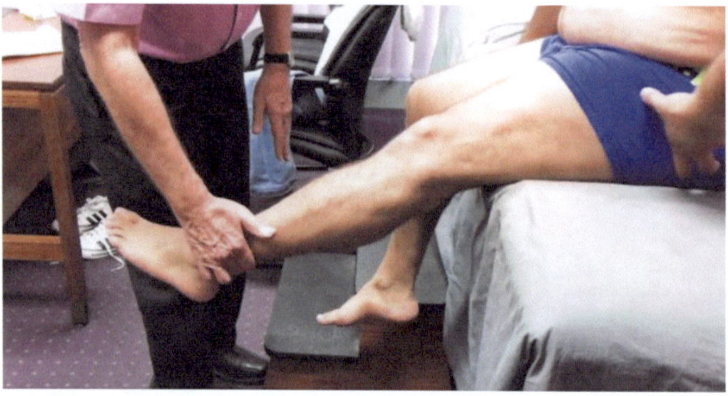

Fig. 10.5 Greater range of SLR in the seated position

10.1.4 Case Study 3

This discrepancy does not only occur in the sitting position but also occurs in the recumbent position when the contralateral hip and knee are flexed.

A 37-year-old male fell three meters from a scaffold in 2020 and sustained an L5 nerve root lesion with sensory loss on the dorsum of his right foot and weakness of extension of his big toe. When examined in 2023, he had significant restriction of SLR on the right side in the supine position (Fig. 10.6) with a significant increase in SLR on the affected side when the contralateral hip and knee are flexed to 90° (Fig. 10.7).

10.1.5 Mechanism

What is the possible mechanism for these observations?

I would like to suggest two hypotheses as to how this phenomenon occurs in cases of radiculopathy or tight hamstrings. It should be noted that the following suggested mechanisms are not applicable in patients who are malingering or who have acute spinal conditions where any movements may be painful.

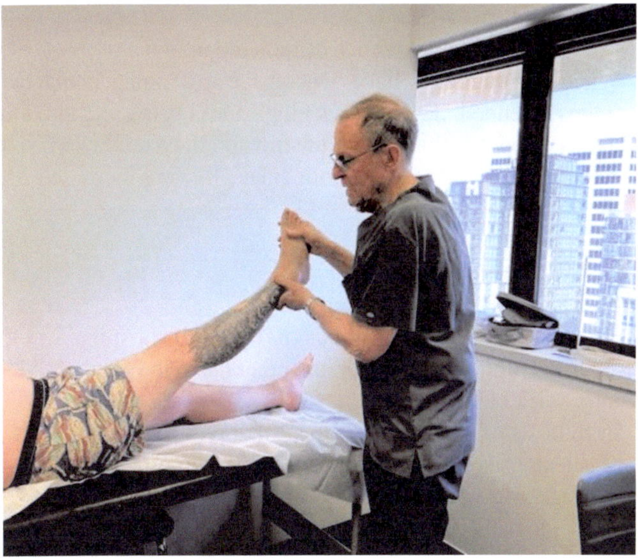

Fig. 10.6 Significant restriction of SLR on the right side in the supine position

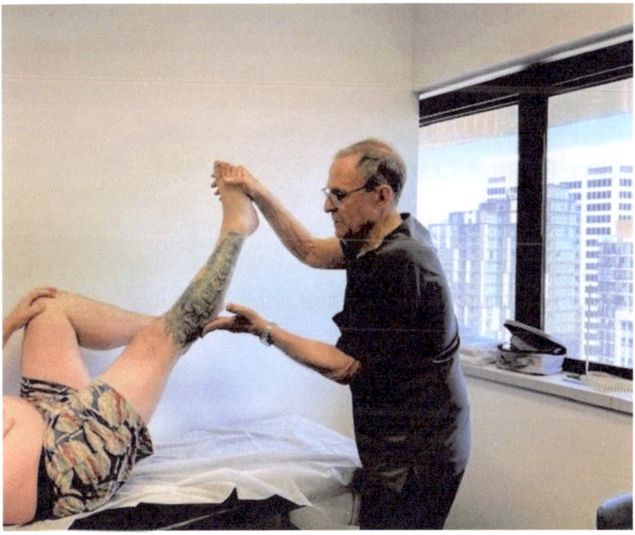

Fig. 10.7 Greater range with contralateral hip and knee flexed

10.1.5.1 Hypothesis 1

Restricted SLR in the presence of radiculopathy.

When the patient is lying flat on the examining couch with both hips extended, the lumbosacral plexus is being anchored in a relatively fixed position. When the hip and knee are flexed, some of the tension is removed on both sides allowing increased SLR on the affected side.

10.1.5.2 Hypothesis 2

Restricted SLR due to tight hamstrings.

Note that in the recumbent position, the lumbar spine is in lordosis. In the sitting position, on the other hand, the spine is able to assume a flexed position.

In lordosis of the lumbar spine, the top of the pelvis tilts forward and the bottom of the pelvis, with the attachment of the hamstrings, tilts backwards, thereby stretching and tightening the origin of the hamstrings. In the flexed position of the lumbar spine (kyphosis), the top of the pelvis tilts backward and the bottom tilts forward, thereby relaxing the tension in the hamstrings and allowing increased SLR. This is readily tested on one's-self. Sit on the edge of a chair, put your heel on the ground with your knee in full extension (Fig. 10.8). Put your lumbar spine in maximal lordosis and test your SLR (Fig. 10.9). Now let your spine flex and note the significant increase in your SLR (Fig. 10.10).

10.1.6 Further Comment

I see the SLR discrepancy so regularly that I cannot imagine that others have not found the same thing. Possibly then we are simply passing on information 'from authority'. Certainly, something to think about!

10.1.7 Conclusion

Straight leg raising in patients with either nerve root involvement (radiculopathy) or tight hamstrings is significantly increased in either the seated position or when the contralateral hip and knee are flexed in the recumbent position. Waddell's distraction test is being misinterpreted to the significant disadvantage of injured workers. An explanation of why this occurs is suggested.

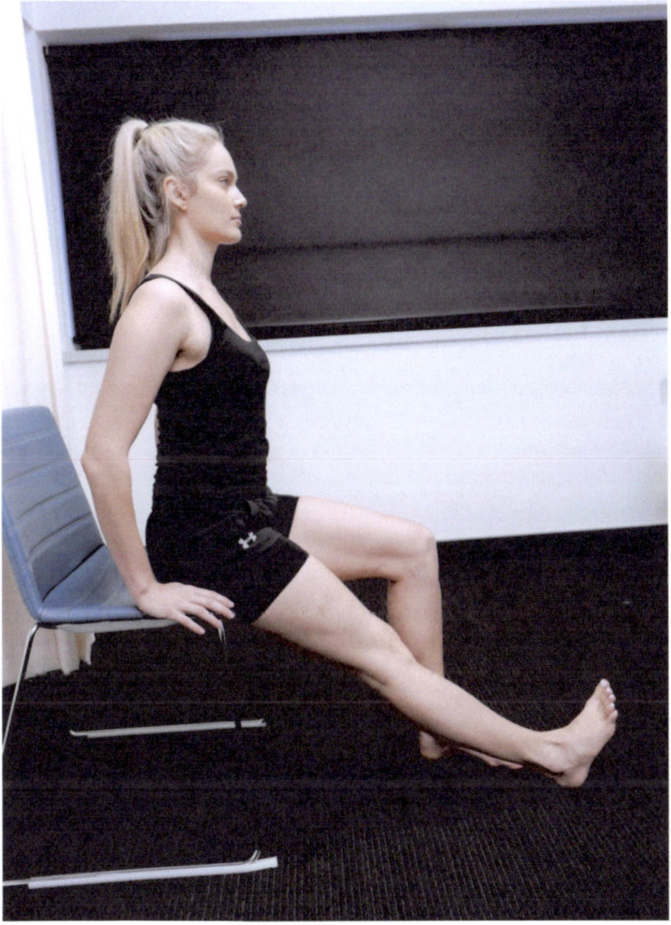

Fig. 10.8 Starting position

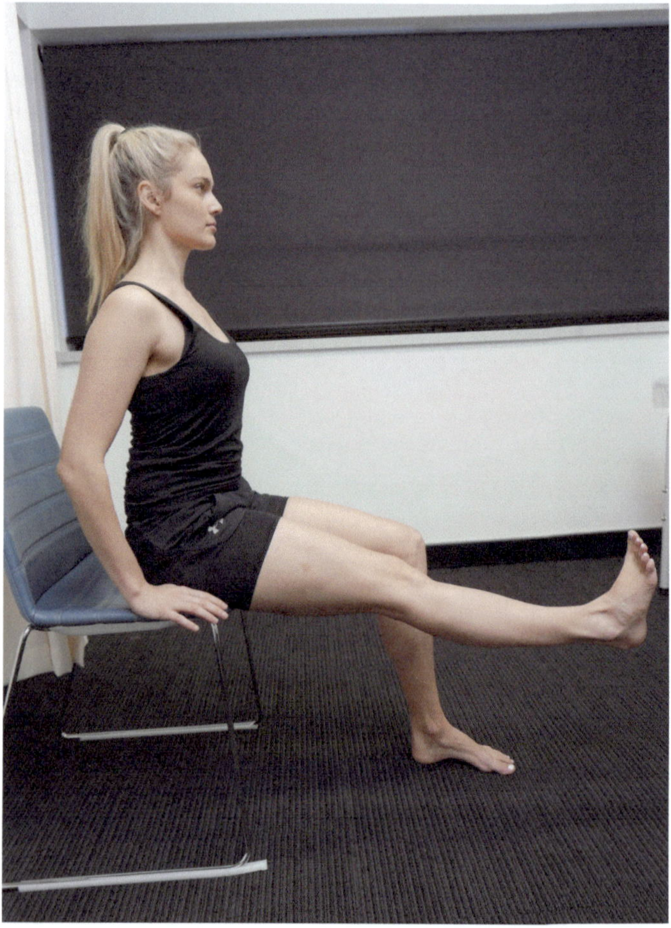

Fig. 10.9 Hamstring tightness lumbar spine in lordosis (extension)

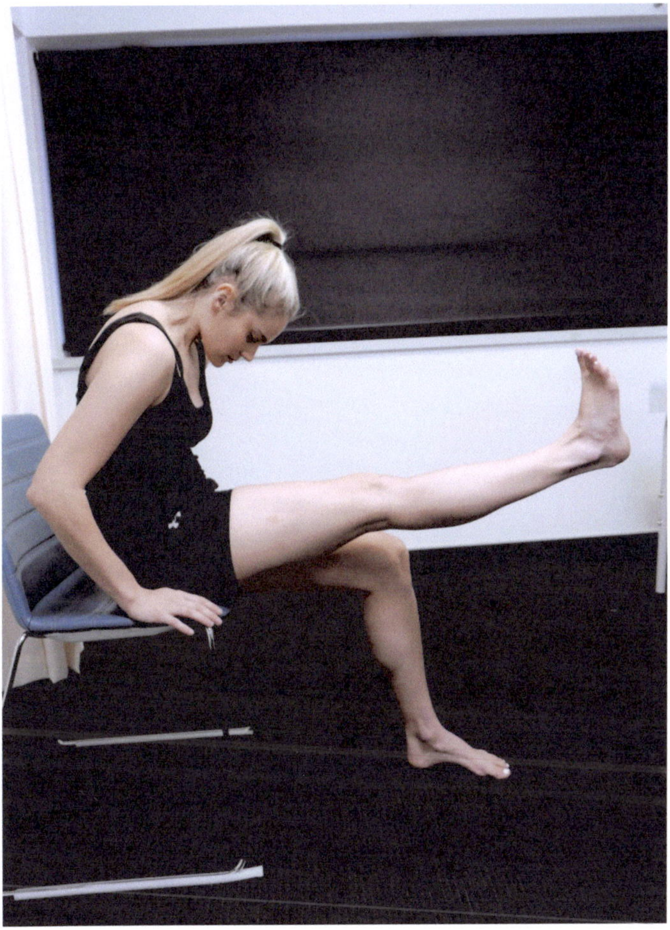

Fig. 10.10 Lumbar spine in flexion

Shortening 11

11.1 Shortening/Leg Length Inequality (LLI)

The usual method used to assess leg length discrepancy is to measure the distance from the anterior superior iliac spine (ASIS) to the tip of the medial malleolus, with the patient supine as shown in Fig. 11.1.

Another method is by using blocks with the patient standing, which is probably more accurate than the supine method. As shown in Fig. 11.2, I use a set of blocks of 0.5, 1, 1.5, and 2 cm. This provides increments of 0.5 cm up to 5 cm. There is also a 5 cm block.

Figure 11.3 illustrates how accurate this method is. Figure 11.3a shows a person with equal leg lengths, and you can see how the fingers placed on the iliac crests are at the same level. In Fig. 11.3b, the right side has been raised on a 1 cm block and you can see the obvious difference in the level of the fingers.

It is sensible to check the measurements using both methods. To get an accurate figure for the amount of shortening, a scanogram is required.

A good method of determining whether the shortening is above or below the knee is to flex the knees to 90° with the feet together on the examining couch:

R. Pillemer, *Physical Signs in Orthopedic and Neurologic Disorders*, https://doi.org/10.1007/978-3-031-99529-3_11

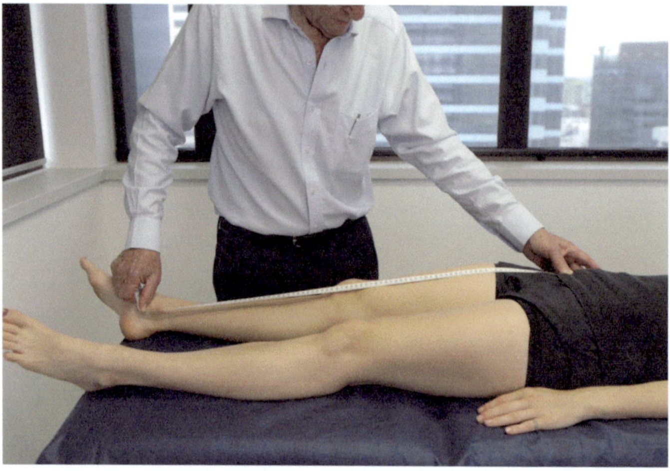

Fig. 11.1 Measuring leg length

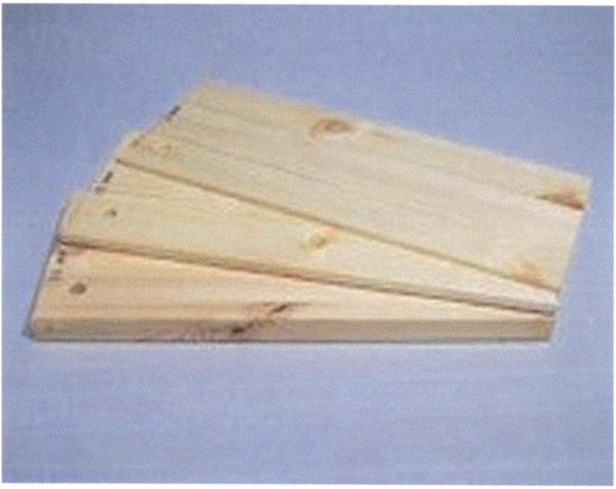

Fig. 11.2 Blocks of varying heights for measuring leg length inequality

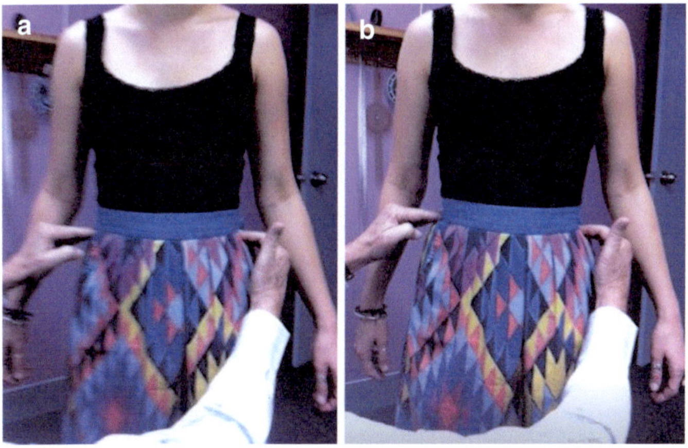

Fig. 11.3 Measuring leg length inequality. (**a**) Fingers on iliac crests and eyes at same level; (**b**) With a 1 cm block on the right side

- The view from the foot of the couch will show tibial shortening (Fig. 11.4a). An inequality in the height of the knees in infants is usually caused by hip dislocation or congenital femoral shortening (positive Galeazzi sign).
- The view from the side will show femoral shortening (Fig. 11.4b).

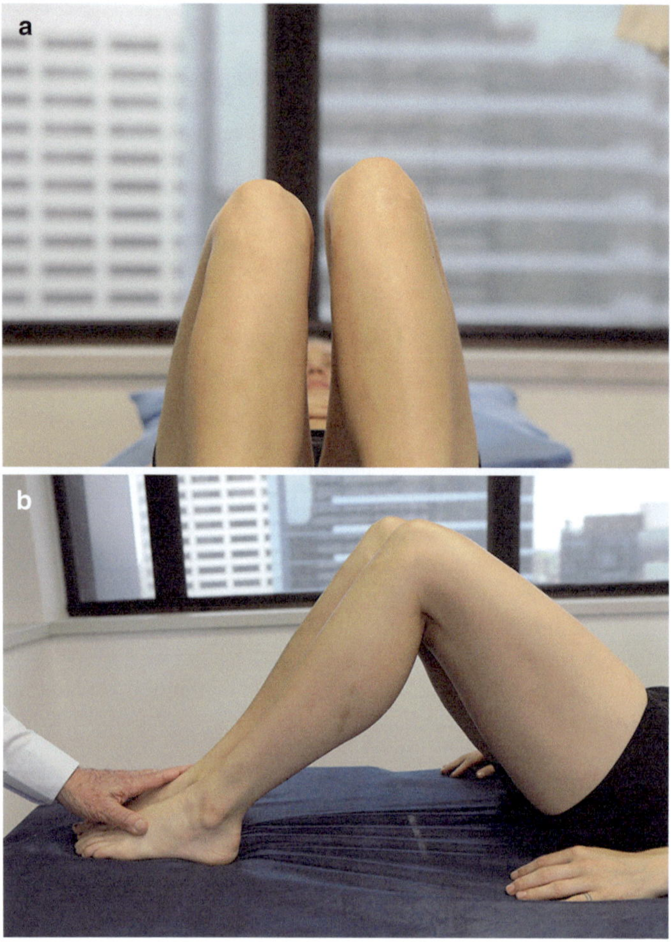

Fig. 11.4 (**a**) Tibial shortening. (**b**) Femoral shortening

11.2 True Versus Apparent Shortening

True shortening means that one leg is indeed shorter than the other. In Fig. 11.5a, the left leg appears shorter than the right leg. True shortening is confirmed if the pelvis is square and the legs are parallel.

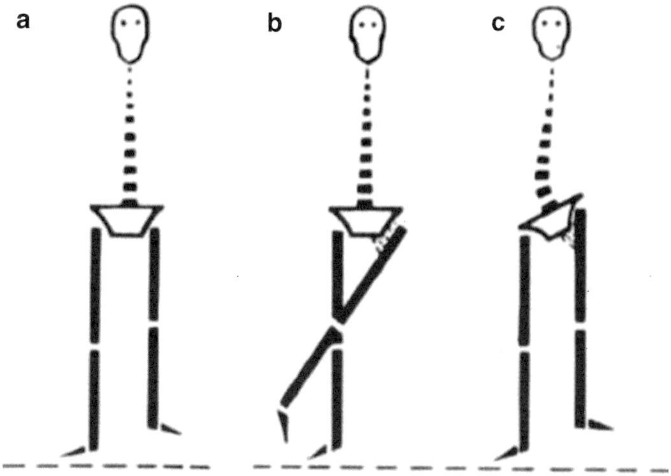

Fig. 11.5 True shortening (**a**) versus apparent shortening (**b**, **c**)

Apparent shortening can be confusing. Figure 11.5b shows an adduction contracture of the left hip, such that when the pelvis is square, the left leg crosses over the right leg. There is no way that the person can walk in this position. The only way that they can get the legs parallel is by hitching up the pelvis on the left side. The person can now walk, and the legs are parallel. The pelvis, however, is not square (Fig. 11.5c). So, the left leg appears to be short even though it is not, and this is called apparent shortening. Note that the person also develops a compensatory scoliosis.

The way to measure apparent shortening is by measuring from a central landmark such as the umbilicus or the xiphisternum to the medial malleolus.

The commonest cause of apparent shortening is an adduction contracture of the hip on the affected side as indicated above and depicted in Fig. 11.6a. Once again, this reveals that to get the legs parallel in order to be able to walk, the pelvis has to be hitched up on the right side, resulting in apparent shortening (Fig. 11.6b).

In Fig. 11.7a, the person has a fixed abduction contracture of the left hip and the only way to get the legs parallel is to hitch up the pelvis on the right side, giving apparent lengthening of the left leg (Fig. 11.7b).

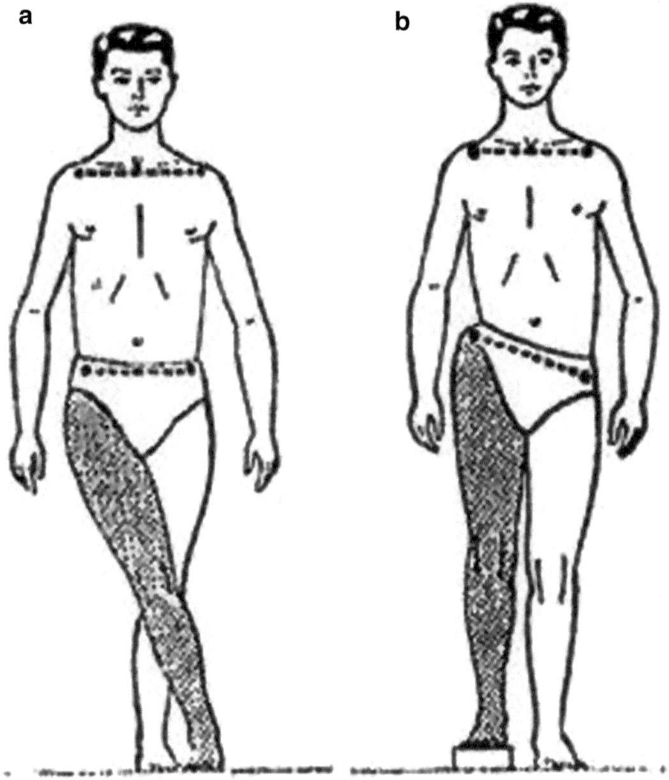

Fig. 11.6 (**a**) Fixed adduction contracture of the right hip; (**b**) resulting apparent shortening

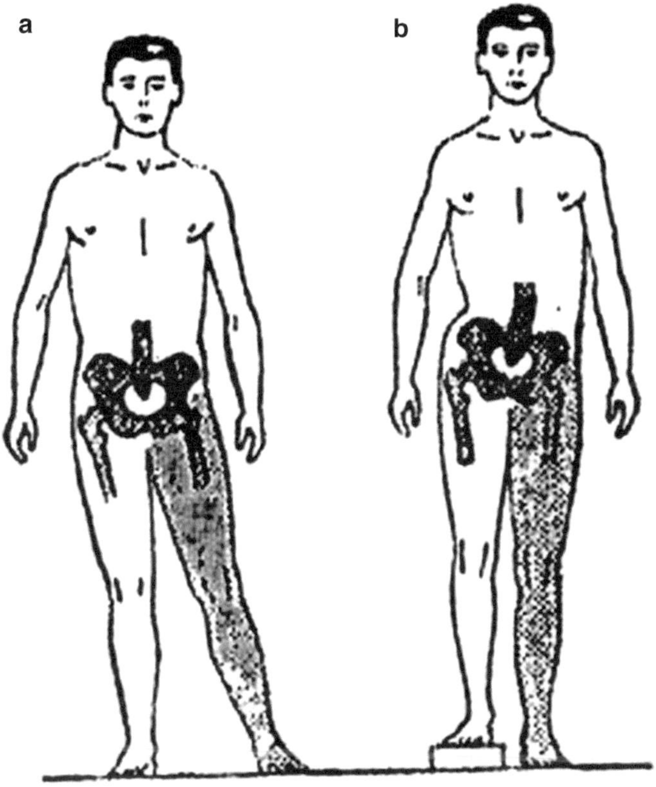

Fig. 11.7 (**a**) Fixed adduction contracture of the left hip; (**b**) resulting apparent lengthening of the left leg

Skeletal Muscle 12

12.1 Some Interesting Observations—Vignettes

The topics will be discussed under the following headings:

A. Overview
B. Muscle contraction
C. Testing motor power
D. Pectoralis major: Isolating the action of the clavicular head
E. Tenodesis and tenodesis effect
F. Latissimus dorsi and teres major: Recall the action
G. Triceps function

12.1.1 Overview

There are three types of muscle:

12.1.1.1 Skeletal Muscle

- Approximately 35% of body weight.
- Under conscious/voluntary control.
- Responsible for skeletal movement.
- Muscle fibres are striated and contain many nuclei.

R. Pillemer, *Physical Signs in Orthopedic and Neurologic Disorders*, https://doi.org/10.1007/978-3-031-99529-3_12

12.1.1.2 Smooth Muscle

- Found in the walls of internal organs
- Under control of autonomic nervous system—involuntary
- Non-striated and have one central nucleus

12.1.1.3 Cardiac Muscle

- Found in the walls of the heart
- Involuntary
- Striated (like skeletal muscle) with one central nucleus (like smooth muscle)

12.1.1.4 Structure of Skeletal Muscle

- See Fig. 12.1.
- Each muscle fibre/cell is enclosed within the endomysium.
- Each bundle of fibres is in turn enclosed within the perimysium.
- The entire muscle is then enclosed within the epimysium.

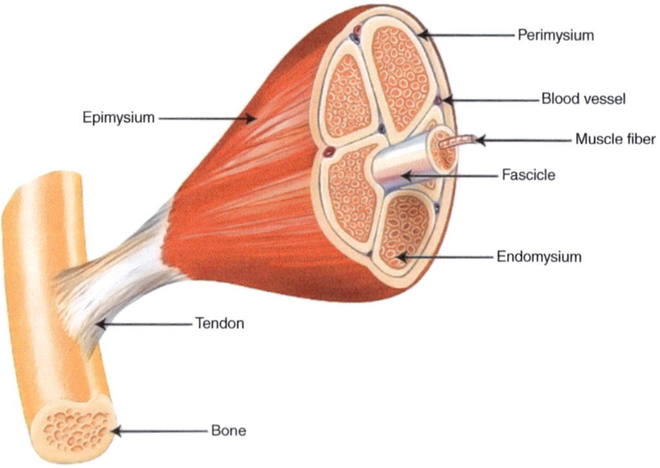

Fig. 12.1 Structure of skeletal muscle

- Muscles attach to bones via tendons at both ends.
- Muscles contract when they receive a nerve impulse.

12.1.2 Muscle Contraction

The type of muscle contraction is determined by the changes in the length of the muscle during contraction.

Consider the example of an arm lifting a heavy weight as in a biceps curl. There are three possibilities (Fig. 12.2):

(i) Concentric contraction: The muscle shortens as the elbow flexes.
(ii) Eccentric contraction: The muscle lengthens as the elbow extends.
(iii) Isometric contraction: There is no change in muscle length and the elbow does not move.

(Note that both concentric and eccentric contractions can be isotonic, that is, where there is constant tension in the muscle as the muscle changes length.)

The example of eccentric contraction[1] in the biceps curl is obvious. Consider also eccentric contraction of the quadriceps muscle when going downstairs. If not for the eccentric quadriceps contraction, the knee would simply collapse. Other examples include running downhill and during exercise, the downward motion of pull-ups or push-ups.

12.1.3 Testing Motor Power

Most of the English-speaking world use various editions of the American Medical Association 'Guides to the Evaluation of Permanent Impairment' (AMA Guides) for the assessment of impairment in workers' compensation and motor accident cases.

[1] Eccentric contraction sounds like a contradiction in terms, as although it is called 'contraction', the muscle is lengthening.

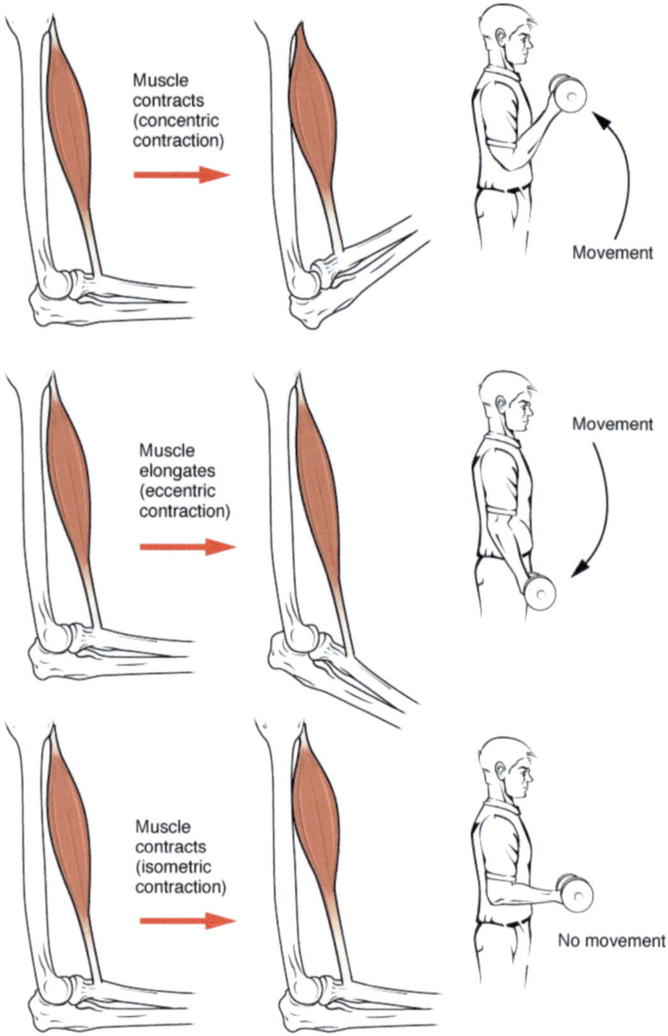

Fig. 12.2 Concentric, eccentric, and isometric contraction

This includes the assessment of 'Motor and Loss-of-Power Deficits Resulting from Peripheral Nerve Disorders Based on Individual Muscle Rating'.

The fourth and fifth editions both have the same six grades, whereas the sixth edition has five grades, similar to the other two. The fifth edition will form the basis for discussion in this section (AMA Fifth Edition: Table 16-11, page 484).

As noted in Fig. 12.3, Grade 5 is normal with 0% motor deficit, while Grade 0 with 'No evidence of contractility' gives 100% motor deficit. This leaves a further four grades, which we will examine individually.

12.1.3.1 Grade 1

'Evidence of slight contractility; no joint movement'. This provides an assessment of between 76% and 99% motor deficit.

Consider

How much useful function is possible with slight muscle contractions, despite no joint movement? Common sense would suggest that there is no useful function and that the motor deficit should be 100%.

12.1.3.2 Grade 2

'Complete active range of motion with gravity eliminated'. This provides an assessment of between 51% and 75% motor deficit.

Consider

Using the wrist as an example, one can flex and extend the wrist with the forearm in mid-rotation with gravity eliminated, but with the forearm in pronation, extension of the wrist is no longer possible. If the range of movement were possible only without gravity, its usefulness would be minimal, if any. The motor deficit should therefore also be 100% or close to 100%.

12.1.3.3 Grade 3

'Complete active range of motion against gravity only, without resistance'. 26–50% motor deficit.

Table 16-11 Determining Impairment of the Upper Extremity Due to Motor and Loss-of-Power Deficits Resulting From Peripheral Nerve Disorders Based on Individual Muscle Rating

a. Classification

Grade	Description of Muscle Function	% Motor Deficit
5	Complete active range of motion against gravity with full resistance	0
4	Complete active range of motion against gravity with some resistance	1- 25
3	Complete active range of motion against gravity only, without resistance	26- 50
2	Complete active range of motion with gravity eliminated	51- 75
1	Evidence of slight contractility; no joint movement	76- 99
0	No evidence of contractility	100

b. Procedure

1	Identify the motion involved, such as flexion, extension, etc.
2	Identify the muscle(s) performing the motion and the motor nerve(s) involved.
3	Grade the severity of motor deficit of individual muscles according to the classification given above.
4	Find the maximum impairment of the upper extremity due to motor deficit for each nerve structure involved: spinal nerves (Table 16-13), brachial plexus (Table 16-14), and major peripheral nerves (Table 16-15).
5	Multiply the severity of the motor deficit by the maximum impairment value to obtain the upper extremity impairment for each structure involved.

Adapted from Lovett RW. From Omer GE Jr. Bell-Krotoski J. Evaluation of clinical results following peripheral nerve suture. In: Omer GE Jr, Spinner M, Van Beek AL, eds. *Management of Peripheral Nerve Problems*. 2nd ed. Philadelphia, Pa: WB Saunders Co; 1998:341; Seddon HJ. *Surgical Disorders of the Peripheral Nerves*. 2nd ed. Edinburgh, Scotland: Churchill Livingstone; 1975; Swanson AB, de Groot Swanson G. Evaluation of permanent impairment in the hand and upper extremity. In: Doege TC, ed. *Guides to the Evaluation of Permanent Impairment*. Fourth ed. Chicago, Ill: American Medical Association; 1993.

Fig. 12.3 Table 16-11 from AMA Fifth Edition, Chapter 16

Consider

A wrist that can actively extend from a position of pronation of the forearm may have some useful function but would not be able to extend while holding anything significant such as a stapler weighing 350 g. Once again common sense would suggest that there would be minimal functional use in such a wrist.

12.1.3.4 Grade 4

'Complete active range of motion against gravity with some resistance'. 1–25% motor deficit.

Discussion

If you agree with the comments made above, about Grades 1–4, it would be appropriate to question how this unfortunate situation came about.

The three references given with Table 16-11 provide the answer. The first is from Seddon HJ 1975, the second from Swanson AB et al. in 1993, and the third from Omer GE Jr 1998 'Evaluation of clinical results following nerve suture'. See Fig. 12.3.

It seems then that what is being measured is the return of motor function after nerve repair and not following nerve injury!

Consider, for example, the patient who has a severe radial nerve in the mid-humeral region, which is repaired primarily. After 3 months, he shows slight contractility of muscles motivating the wrist but with no joint movement (Grade 1). While the surgeon and the patient may well be delighted with the result, there is obviously no useful function present. The Guides only allow 76–99% motor deficit.

After a further 2 months, the patient may demonstrate active movement of the wrist with gravity eliminated (Grade 2) and therefore still minimal if any useful function. According to the Guides, this would be associated with only 51–75% motor deficit.

Grades 3 and 4 would demonstrate progress with regard to nerve recovery with minimal useful function in early Grade 3 to almost normal function in late Grade 4.

12.1.3.5 Conclusion

A far more useful and accurate assessment of motor deficit, as well as being more beneficial to the patient, is suggested in

	Mild	Moderate	Severe
Motor weakness	1 - 33	34 - 66	67 - 100
Range of motion of affected joint/joints	1 - 33	34 - 66	67 - 100
Muscle wasting	1 - 33	34 - 66	67 - 100

Fig. 12.4 Guidance for assessing percentage motor deficit

Fig. 12.4. The figures of impairment suggested are equivalent to Grades 3 and 4 in AMA 5 (which encompass minimal return of function to near normal return of function). Impairment would range between 1% and 99%.

Criteria to consider would include the extent of the motor weakness and the resulting loss of range of movement of the affected joint/joints. The extent of muscle wasting would also be a relevant objective clinical finding.

While this method could potentially result in a wide range of opinions, a consistent result could be anticipated from physicians with clinical experience, some guidelines, and an open mind.

Considering the most relevant clinical findings, a decision could therefore be made to select the appropriate percentage of impairment.

12.1.4 Pectoralis Major: Isolating the Action of the Clavicular Head

The largest muscle of the anterior chest wall with two heads, sternocostal and clavicular, which converge on the upper humerus and form the anterior wall of the axilla (Fig. 12.5).

12.1.4.1 Origin

The sternocostal head arises from:

- The anterior surface of the manubrium and body of the sternum
- The anterior surface of the superior six costal cartilages
- The superior part of the aponeurosis of external oblique

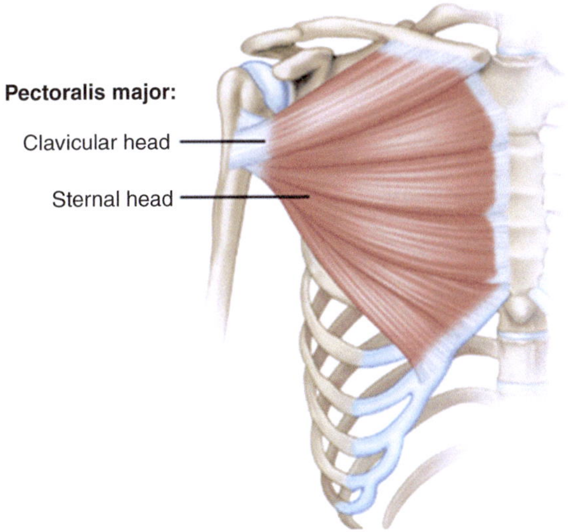

Fig. 12.5 Pectoralis major

The clavicular head arises from:

- The anterior surface of the medial half of the clavicle

12.1.4.2 Insertion

- The tendon is inserted into the lateral lip of the bicipital groove.
- Note that the tendon folds on itself in the axilla such that the lower fibres insert higher on the humerus than the upper fibres from the clavicular head (Fig. 12.6).

12.1.4.3 Nerve Supply

See Fig. 12.7.

The sternocostal head: from the medial cord of the brachial plexus via the medial pectoral nerve (C6,7,8 and T1).

The clavicular head: From the lateral cord of the brachial plexus via the lateral pectoral nerve (C5,6).

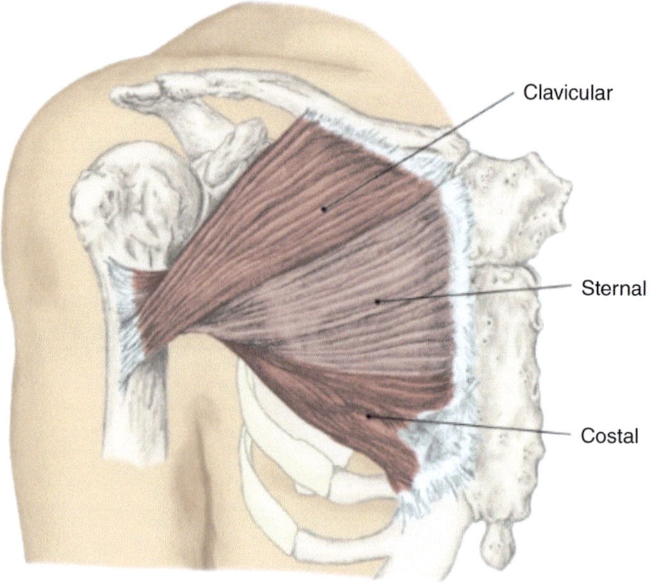

Fig. 12.6 Anterior view identifying the three segments of pectoralis major

12.1.4.4 Isolating the Action of the Clavicular Head

Pectoralis major adducts and medially rotates the arm at the glenohumeral joint. Above 90° of abduction of the shoulder, the clavicular head transversely adducts the arm.

The two heads are clearly visible when adducting the arm against resistance below 90° (Fig. 12.8).

To demonstrate the isolated function of the clavicular head, the actions of the sternocostal head are de-functioned by abducting and externally rotating the arm above 90°, the functions opposite to those of the sternocostal head.

With the shoulder maintained in this position (abduction and external rotation), the palm of the hand is pressed firmly against the side of the head above the ear. The clavicular head will be seen to contract in isolation (Fig. 12.9), while the sternoclavicular head remains flaccid (Fig. 12.10).

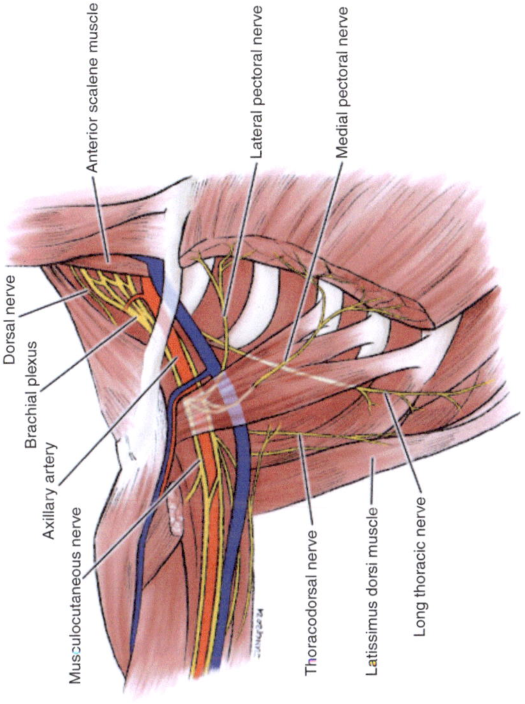

Fig. 12.7 The lateral and medial pectoral nerve

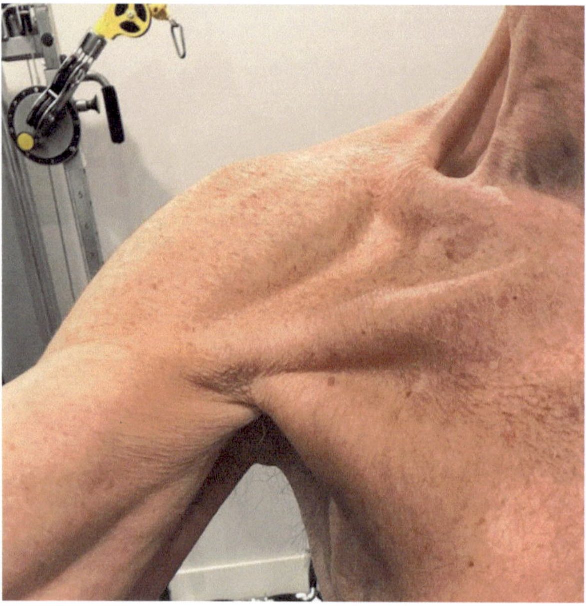

Fig. 12.8 The two heads of pectoralis major clearly visible when adducting arm against resistance below 90°.

12.1.5 Tenodesis and Tenodesis Effect

12.1.5.1 Tenodesis

The operation of suturing the end of a tendon to a bone (Merriam-Webster 2024).

The commonest use of the term is in relation to biceps tenodesis where the damaged section of the biceps tendon is resected, and the remaining tendon is then reattached to the upper humerus by way of screw fixation or endobutton technique (Fig. 12.11).

It is interesting to note that a rotator cuff repair is in fact a tenodesis, when the cuff is sutured to bone in the usual form of repair (Fig. 12.12). Other techniques are also available such as repair of partial tears (intrasubstance repairs) or using a patch to fill a defect.

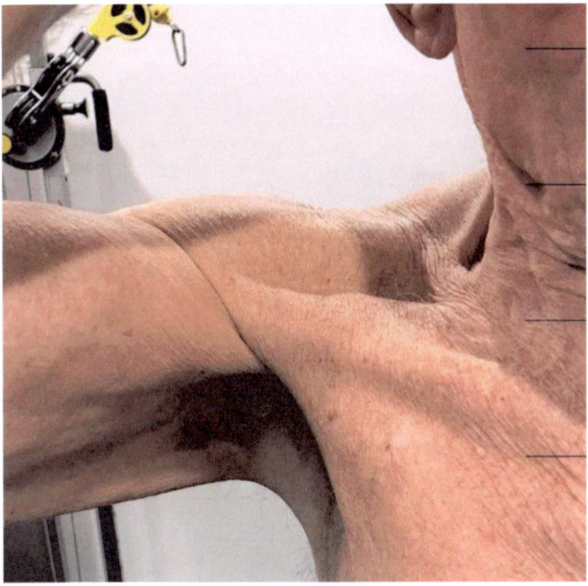

Fig. 12.9 Contraction of the clavicular head in isolation.

Tenodesis is used routinely in hand surgery, for example:

- In flexor digitorum profundus (FDP) injuries, with an intact flexor digitorum superficialis (FDS), the distal section of FDP is sutured to the flexor synovial sheath over the middle phalanx, preventing hyperextension of the DIPJ while allowing passive flexion.
- In the Zancolli lasso procedure (ZLP), the cut end of the FDS donor tendon is wrapped around the FDP A1 pulley (Fig. 12.13) of the affected digits and sutured to itself, thus preventing hyperextension of the MP joint. As noted in Fig. 12.14, the FDS tendon can also be sutured to the lateral band or to bone (tenodesis).
- In radial nerve, palsy tenodesis of extensor digitorum communis (EDC) to the dorsal surface of the radius will cause extension of the MCP joints with active or passive wrist flexion.

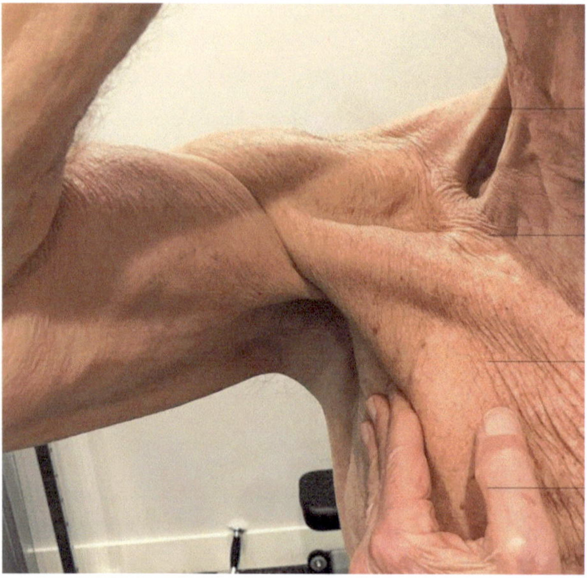

Fig. 12.10 Sternoclavicular head remains flaccid

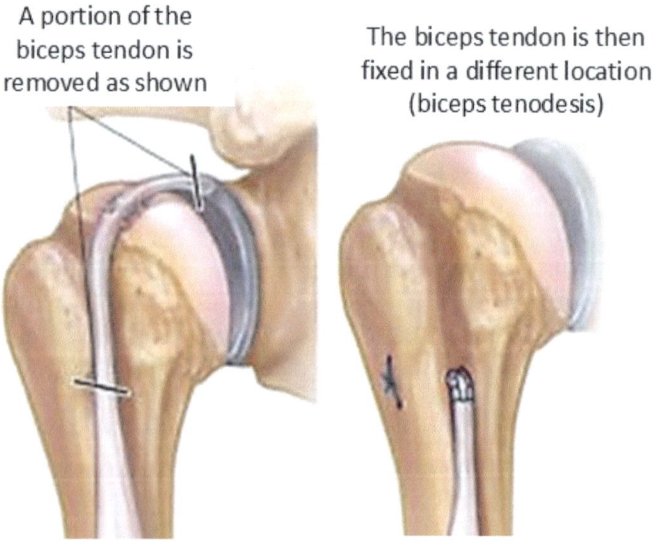

Fig. 12.11 Biceps tenodesis

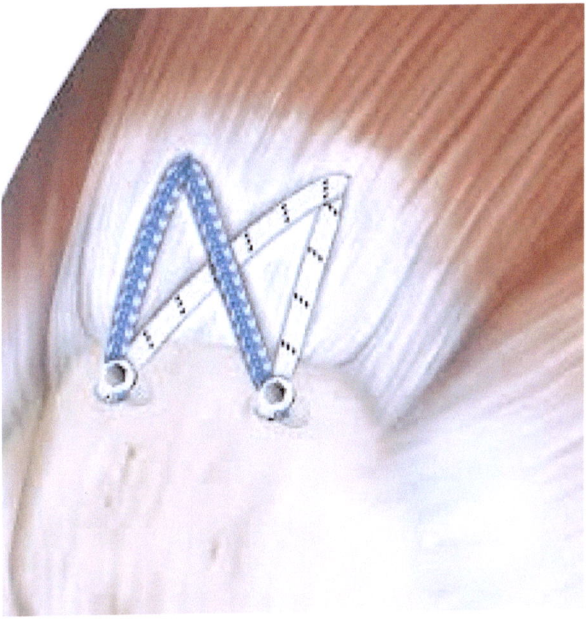

Fig. 12.12 Knotless rotator cuff repair

12.1.5.2 Tenodesis Effect

This is a normal physiological process whereby joint motion of a proximal joint causes synchronous movement of neighbouring joints.

This is most readily observed in relation to the wrist, whereby active extension of the wrist is accompanied by passive flexion of the fingers (1), while active flexion of the wrist is accompanied by passive extension of the fingers (2) (Fig. 12.15).

(1) Due to tightening/relative shortening of the flexor tendons
(2) Due to tightening/relative shortening of the extensor tendons

This function is particularly useful in cases of spinal cord injury with quadriplegia at the C6 level, where there is still active wrist extension but no active finger flexion. With active rehabilitation, patients can be taught to optimise this tenodesis effect and develop a passive whole hand grasp with relative shortening of the

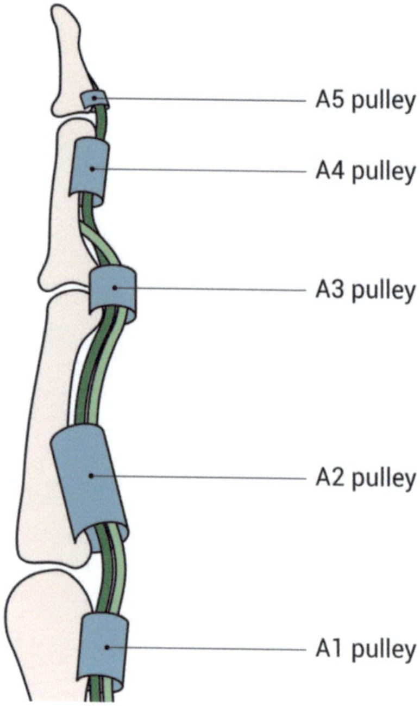

Fig. 12.13 Flexor pulleys of the finger

finger flexors (Fig. 12.16), as well as passive lateral grip due to shortening of flexor pollicis longus (Fig. 12.17).

The tenodesis effect is also especially useful in examination of the hand regarding diagnosis. For example, in flexor tendon injuries, the involved finger will not go into flexion with extension of the wrist but will remain extended (Fig. 12.18).

In the Bunnell test for intrinsic tightness, passive extension of the MP joint will result in limited active or passive PIP joint flexion with normal PIP joint flexion with the MP joint in flexion (Fig. 12.19).

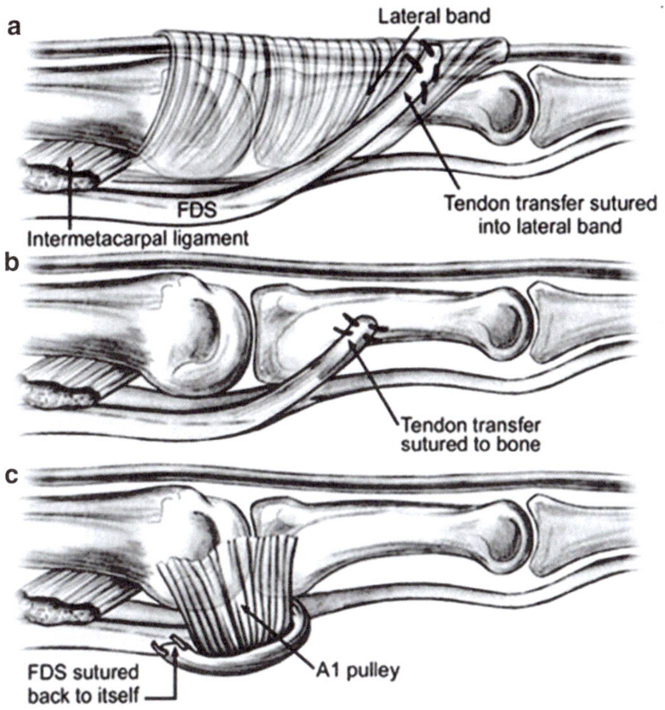

Fig. 12.14 Zancolli lasso procedure (ZLP): three methods

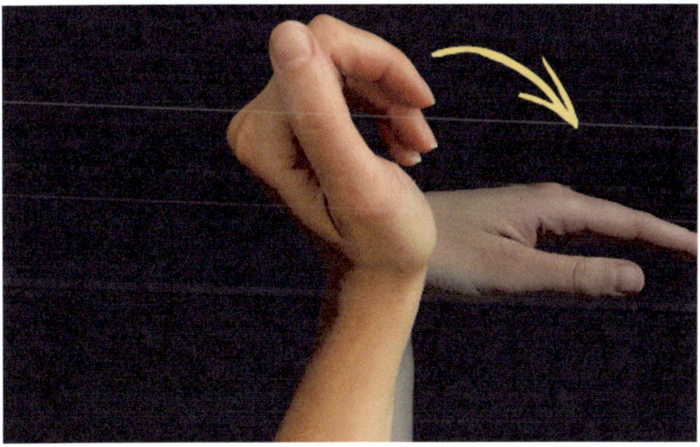

Fig. 12.15 Active extension and flexion of the wrist

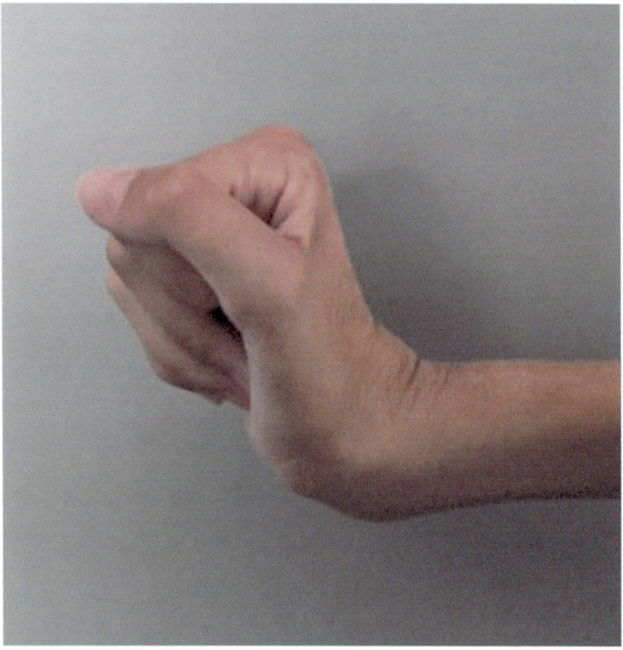

Fig. 12.16 Tenodesis effect

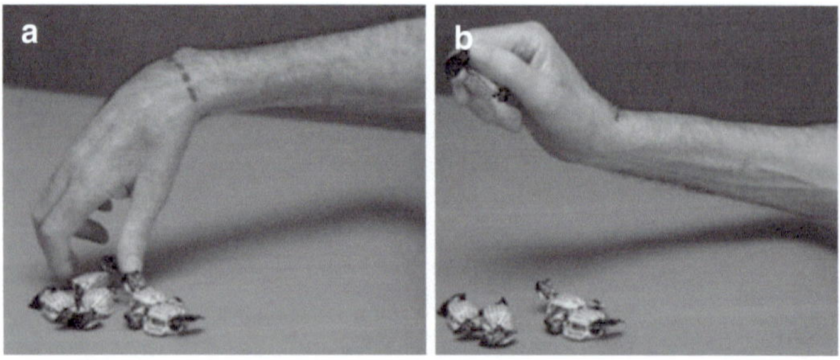

Fig. 12.17 Passive lateral grip due to shortening of flexor pollicis longus (FPL): (**a**) wrist in flexion. (**b**) wrist in extension with passive lateral grip due to shortening of flexor pollicis longus

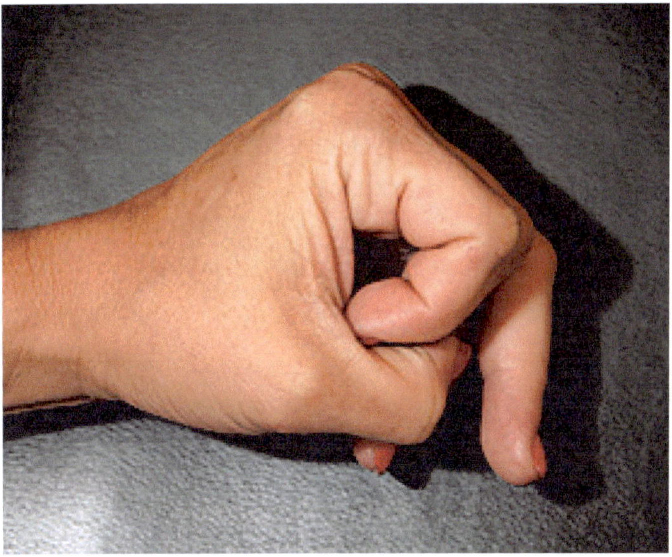

Fig. 12.18 Flexor tendon injury

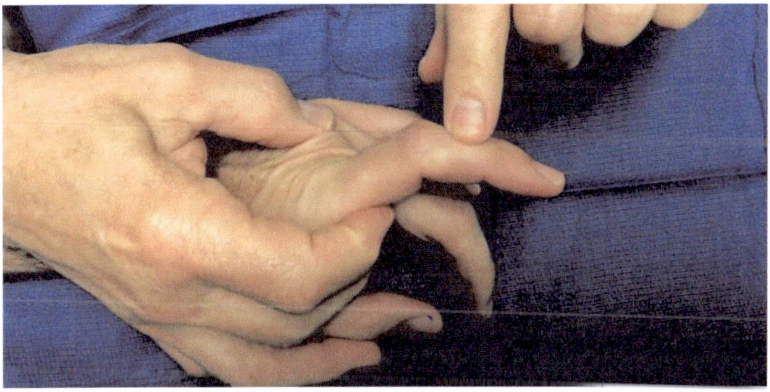

Fig. 12.19 Bunnell test for intrinsic tightness

12.1.6 Latissimus Dorsi and Teres Major

'Recall the function'

Both muscles have a similar function in relation to the shoulder. If one visualises the origin and insertion, the actions are:

- Internal rotation
- Extension
- Adduction

12.1.6.1 Latissimus Dorsi

Origin

- See Fig. 12.20
- Lower 6 thoracic vertebral spinous processes

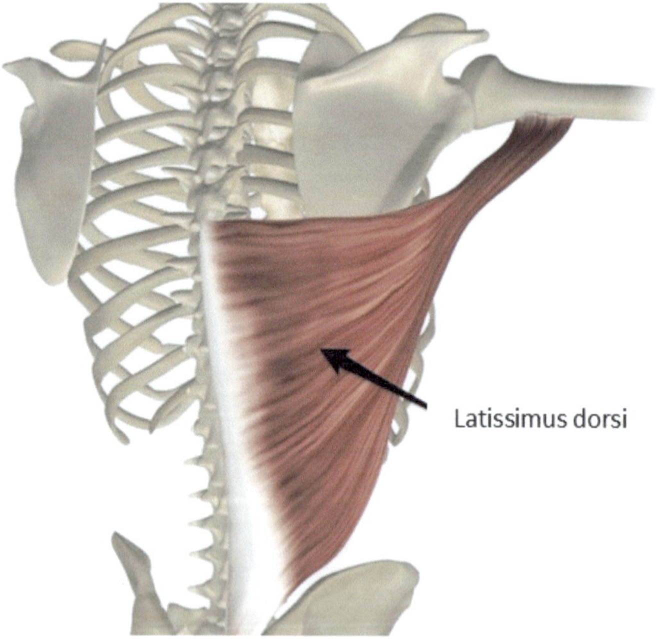

Fig. 12.20 Latissimus dorsi

- Lumbar and sacral spinous processes (T6–S5) through the thoracolumbar fascia and supraspinous ligament
- Posterior iliac crest and lower four ribs, and the inferior angle of the scapula

Insertion

- As a flat tendon on the floor of the bicipital (intertubercular) groove of the humerus (Fig. 12.21)

Innervation

- Thoracodorsal nerve (C6–C8) from the posterior cord of the brachial plexus

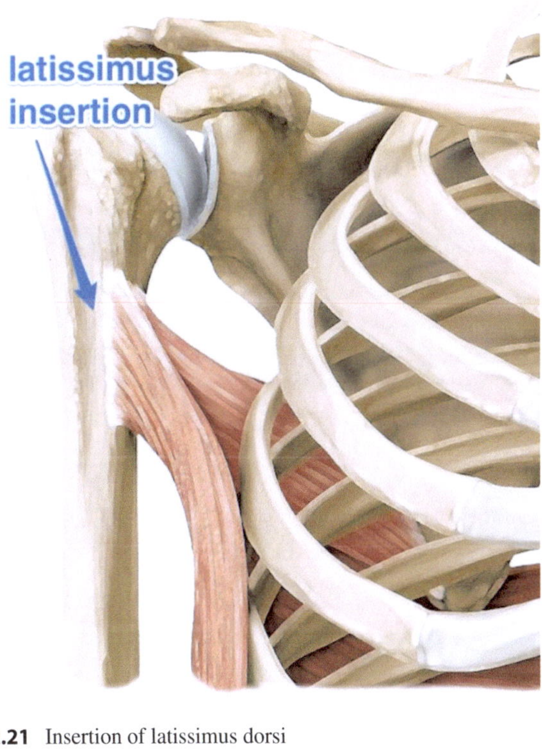

Fig. 12.21 Insertion of latissimus dorsi

12.1.6.2 Teres Major

Origin

- Dorsal surface of the inferior angle of the scapula (Fig. 12.22)

Insertion

- The medial lip of the bicipital (intertubercular) groove of the humerus (Figs. 12.21 and 12.23)

Innervation

- Lower subscapular nerve (C5, C6)

Recalling the function of latissimus dorsi and teres major:

Place the dorsum of your hand on your sacrum (Fig. 12.24f). In order to get here from the anatomical position (Fig. 12.24a), internally rotate the arm (Fig. 12.24b), extend from this position

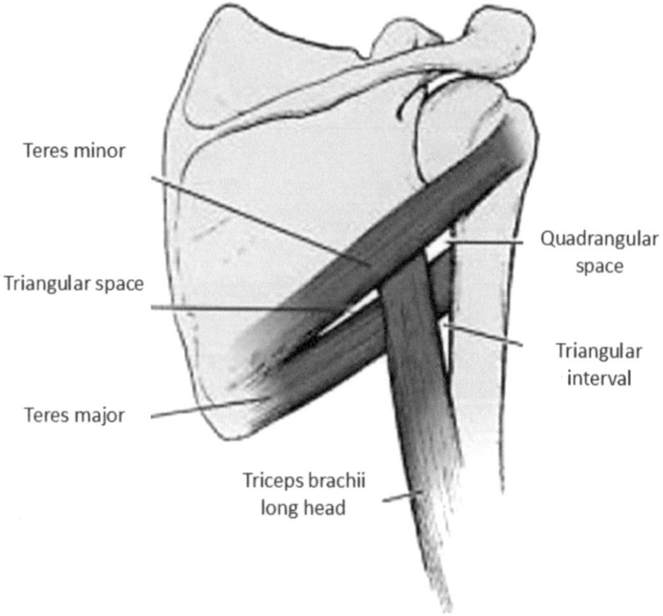

Fig. 12.22 Origin of teres major

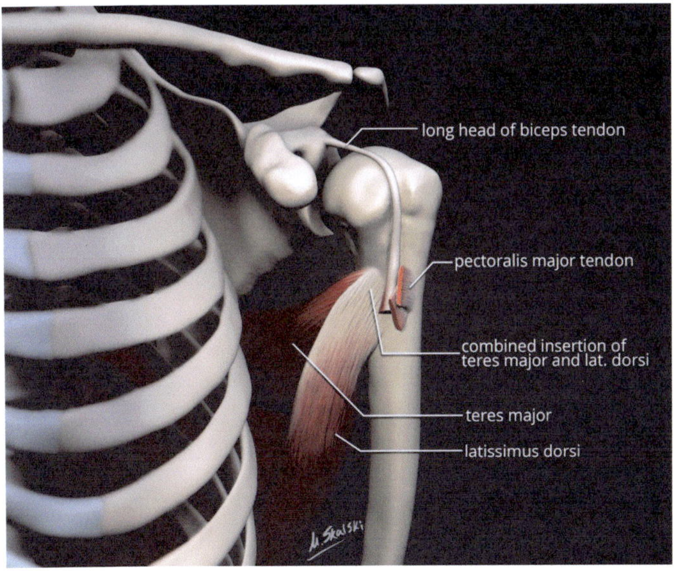

Fig. 12.23 Insertion of teres major

(Fig. 12.24c, d), then adduct to reach the sacrum (Fig. 12.24e, f). That is, internal rotation, extension, and adduction.

Note: Latissimus dorsi is the 'climbing muscle'; that is, when the arm is fixed above the head as in climbing or doing chin-ups, it will lift the trunk.

12.1.7 Triceps Brachii with Some Interesting Observations

Triceps brachii (TB) is the only muscle in the posterior compartment of the arm. It has three heads (Fig. 12.25): long (red), lateral (yellow), and medial (green), with the medial head lying deep to the other heads.

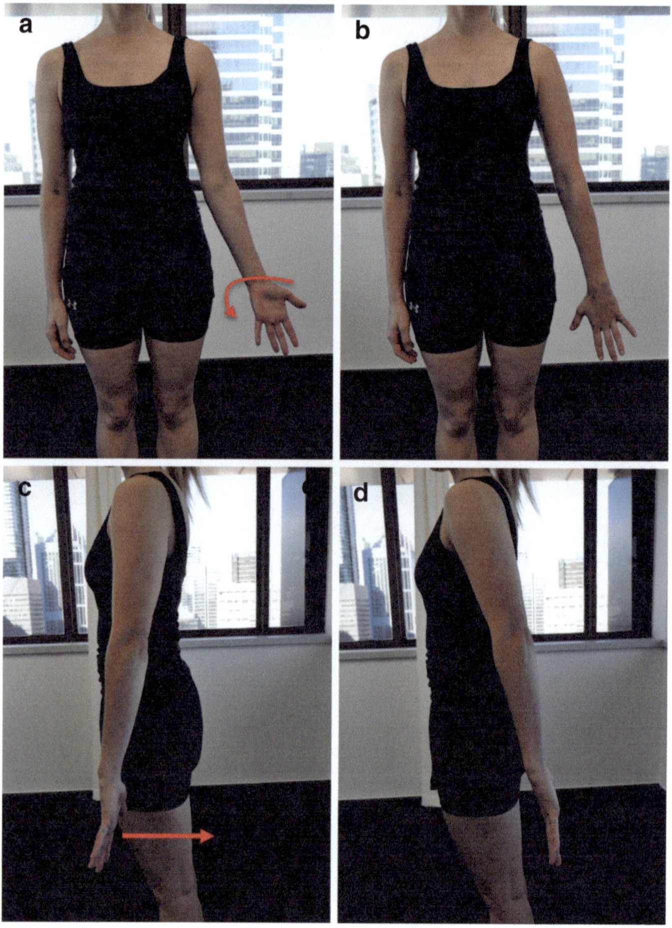

Fig. 12.24 Internal rotation, extension, and adduction; (**a**) anatomical position; (**b**) internal rotation of arm; (**c**) extension of arm to (**d**); (**e**) adduction from the extended position to reach the sacrum; (**f**) final position – dorsum of hand on sacrum

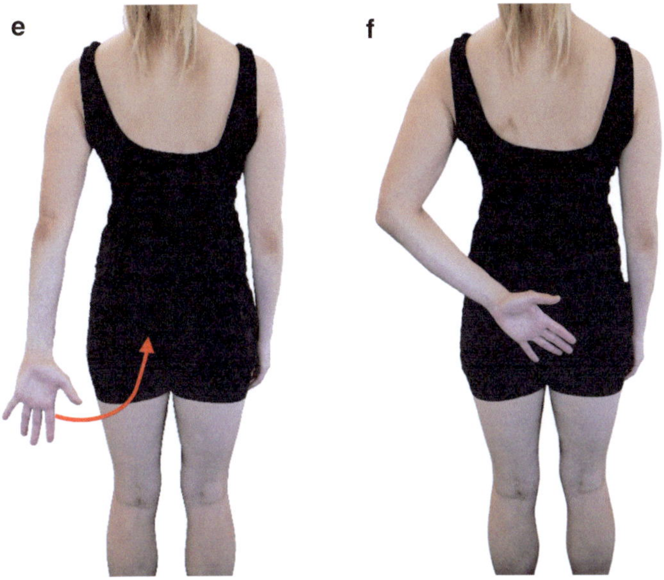

Fig. 12.24 (continued)

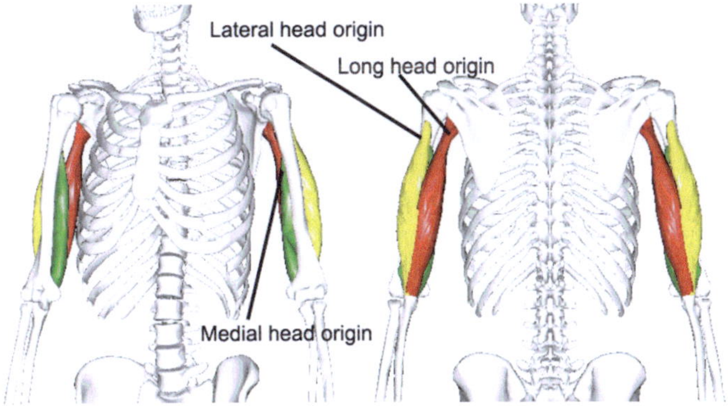

Fig. 12.25 Three heads of triceps brachii

Origin

- Long head: Infra-glenoid tubercle of the scapula (Fig. 12.26)
- Lateral head: Posterior aspect of the humerus, superior to the radial groove (Fig. 12.28)
- Medial head: Posterior aspect of the humerus (Fig. 12.27), inferior to the radial groove (Fig. 12.28)

Insertion

- Posterior surface of the olecranon

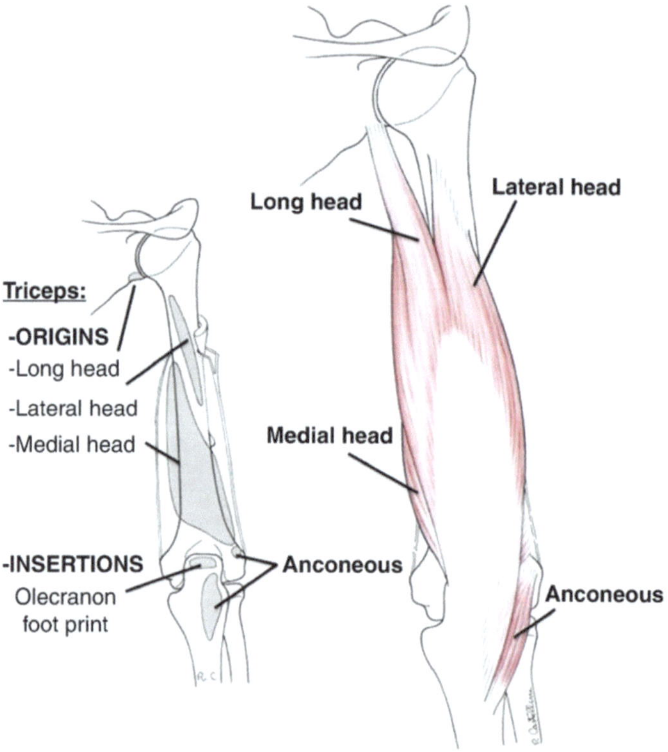

Fig. 12.26 Origin of long head of triceps brachii

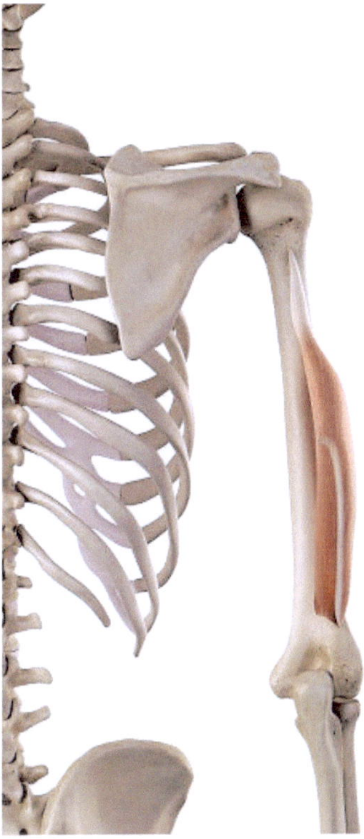

Fig. 12.27 Origin of the medial head of triceps brachii

Nerve Supply

- Radial nerve (C7,8) (Fig. 12.29)

Action

Extension of the forearm/elbow joint.

12.1.7.1 Some Interesting Observations

It is worth considering under what circumstances we do use triceps in everyday activities, that is, with active extension of the elbow. We use our triceps in circumstances such as pressing down on a chair or table when getting up from a seated position particularly associated with a sore back, hip, or knee, also, when doing push-ups, using crutches, or propelling a wheelchair.

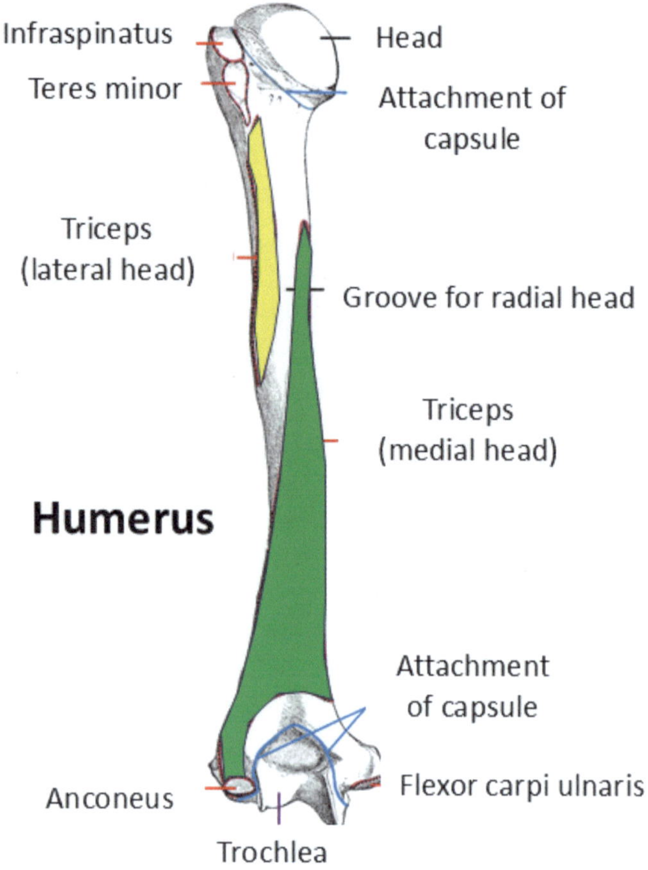

Fig. 12.28 Humerus showing origins of medial and lateral heads of triceps

But when else do we use our triceps? I saw a lady who had suffered an avulsion of her triceps which for several reasons had not been repaired. At the time of examination, she had no active extension of her elbow. She told me that there were only two things that she was aware of that she was unable to do. Use her hair dryer as it would simply drop on her head and (surprisingly) cut food! Think about it, both of these activities clearly require active use of the triceps.

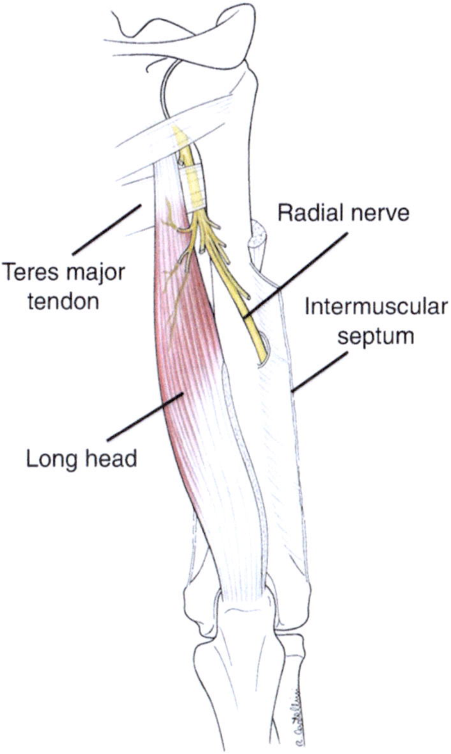

Fig. 12.29 Anatomy of the radial nerve

We do not use triceps when we are putting a heavy weight down on to a surface as this is achieved by eccentric contraction of the biceps (see page 153 (section 12.1.2)). Extending the elbow from a flexed position without any weight, as after touching one's face, is by gravity, again assisted by biceps.

Consider this question regarding triceps function. A patient needs to use a crutch on his right side to be able walk but has a non-functioning triceps on that side. How could they overcome this problem?

By using a long staff with the shoulder in elevation and using the elbow flexors (biceps, brachialis, and brachioradialis) for power, one can keep the elbow in extension despite the absence of triceps function by gripping the staff with the long flexors and extensors of wrist and fingers.

One of the golden rules of skeletal muscle activity is that 'All skeletal muscles can only pull; they never push'. How does this apply when one does a 'push-up'? This is using triceps, and the overall effect is certainly one of pushing. The triceps however is shortening, that is, 'pulling'.

Joints Tidbits 13

13.1 Upper Extremity

13.1.1 Shoulder Joint

13.1.1.1 Physical Signs of Anterior Dislocation of the Shoulder

Several physical signs have been described in anterior shoulder dislocation including the following:

- Prominence of the acromion, the most obvious finding.
- Loss of the rounded shape of the shoulder and loss of deltoid contour.
- Slight external rotation of the arm.
- The patient tends to lean towards the injured side.
- The inability to move the joint associated with intense pain.
- Prominence of the humeral head anteriorly with a void posteriorly.

I would like to suggest another sign which I have not seen described previously, which is present in every case and is clearly visible.

In patients with anterior shoulder dislocation, there appears to be lateral angulation of the distal arm relative to the proximal arm, with the apparent angulation being slightly above the centre of the

R. Pillemer, *Physical Signs in Orthopedic and Neurologic Disorders*, https://doi.org/10.1007/978-3-031-99529-3_13

arm (Fig. 13.1). Not only does the head of the humerus displace anteriorly and inferiorly, but also medially, and the whole shaft of the humerus inclines laterally. This is evident in the distal arm but masked by the prominent acromion and deltoid in the proximal arm, hence the appearance of angulation.

13.1.2 Elbow Joint

13.1.2.1 Malunited Supracondylar Fracture of the Humerus

The following is noted when testing the range of movement of the elbow joint in a patient with a healed malunited supracondylar fracture of the humerus where the supracondylar fragment is displaced more posteriorly on the medial side than the lateral side and tilted more proximally on the medial side.

With the elbow flexed to 90°, there is found to be an increased range of supination compared to the opposite side. When tested with the elbow fully extended, there is found to be an increased range of pronation compared to the opposite side.

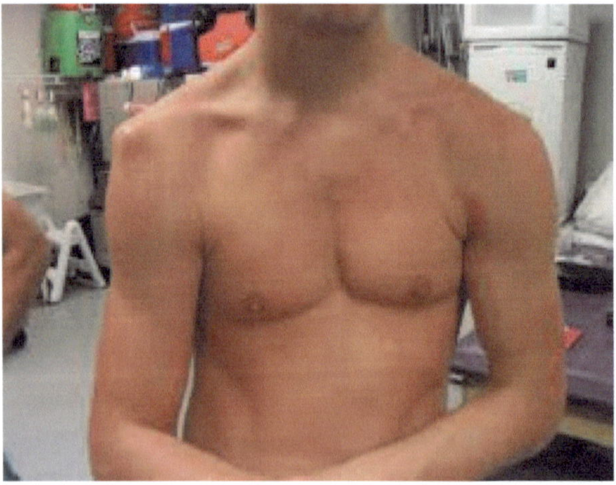

Fig. 13.1 Apparent lateral angulation of the distal arm in anterior dislocation of the shoulder

In summary, there is increased supination in flexion and increased pronation in extension. Taking into account the displacements suggested above, try and picture why this is the case.

13.1.2.2 Explanation

With the elbow flexed to 90° and the thumb pointing to the roof (Fig. 13.2), proximal tilting of the medial side will result in increased supination of the forearm in the coronal plane (Fig. 13.3).

With the elbow in extension, the greater posterior rotation of the medial rather than the lateral aspect of the fragment will allow increased pronation of the forearm in the sagittal plane (Fig. 13.4).

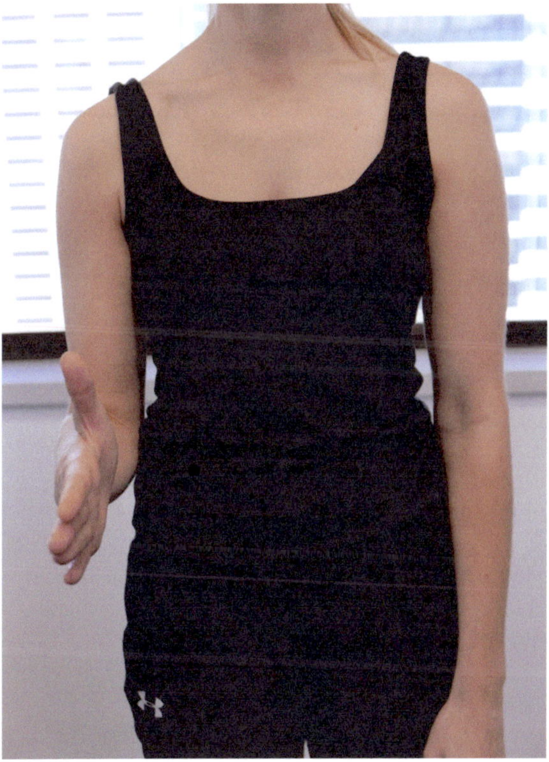

Fig. 13.2 Neutral position

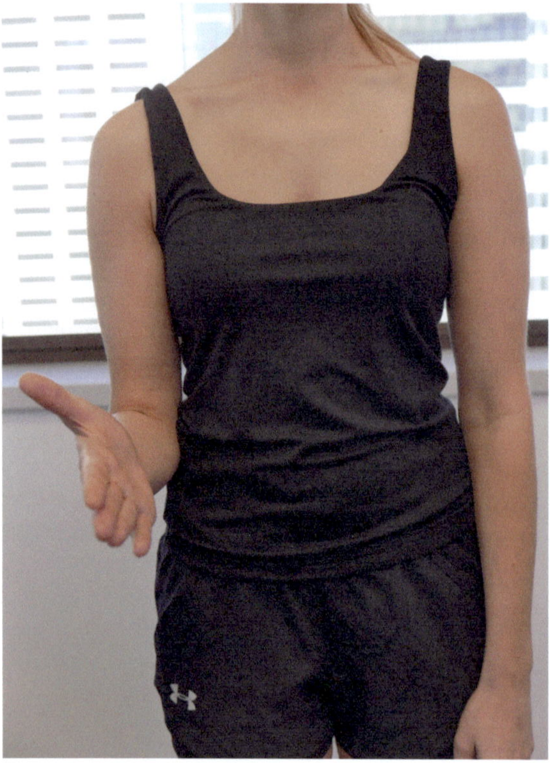

Fig. 13.3 Increased supination

13.1.2.3 Pronation Versus Supination

Here is something to think about regarding the relative importance of pronation versus supination.

- Say for example, you had lost half of either movement and had been left with only 45° of either pronation or supination. Which would you choose?

Suggestion

- If you have only 45° of supination of your forearm, there is no way that you can apply shaving cream or moisturizer to your

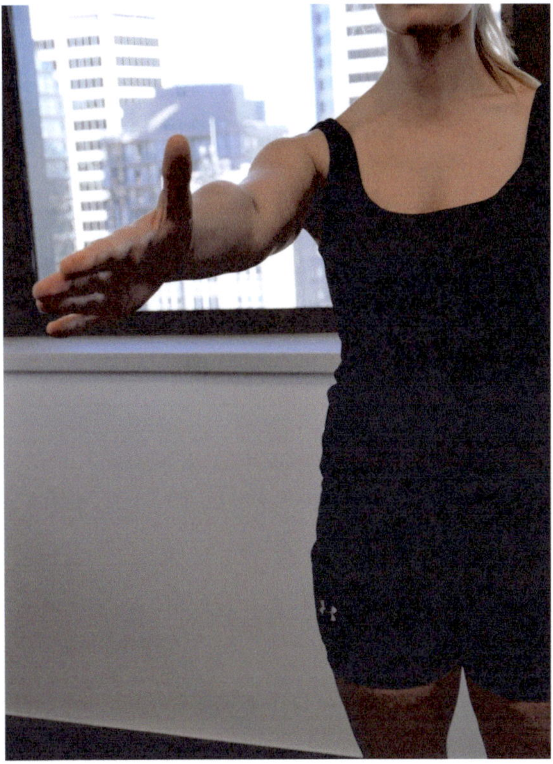

Fig. 13.4 Increased pronation

opposite cheek, you cannot accept coins as change and while you can get your hand to your perineum, you cannot wipe!

- Loss of supination is therefore a very significant disability as there is no way that you can get your hand into a fully supinated position and your body gets in the way when you attempt to do so.
- On the other hand, if you only have 45° of pronation, to get your hand into a fully pronated position, all you need to do is abduct your shoulder to 45°.
- And if you are seated and you want to place your hand flat on the table, just add a bit of internal rotation of your shoulder.

(It is interesting to note that AMA 5 awards more impairment for loss of pronation than for the equivalent loss of supination).

13.1.3 Wrist Joint

As noted in the chapter on 'Skeletal Muscle', active extension of the wrist is accompanied by passive flexion of the fingers, while active flexion of the wrist is accompanied by passive extension of the fingers. This function is particularly useful in cases of spinal cord injury with quadriplegia at the C6 level where patients with no functioning finger flexion can be taught to develop functioning hands because of this tenodesis effect (See Sect. 12.1.5.2, page 165).

It is also worth noting that in active use of the wrist, extension is combined with radial abduction as in gripping firmly, while flexion is combined with ulnar adduction,[1] for example, when hammering in a nail.

13.1.4 Metacarpophalangeal (MP) Joints

Important considerations:

- The heads of the metacarpals are cam shaped so that the distance from centre of the metacarpal head to its palmar articular surface is longer than to the distal articular surface (Fig. 13.5).
- Therefore, when the MP joint is in extension, the collateral ligaments are relatively loose, whereas at 90° of flexion the ligaments tighten because of the cam effect.
- Any prolonged immobilisation in the extended position can lead to shortening and contracture of the collateral ligaments. Immobilisation of the MP joints should therefore always be in flexion.[2]

---

[1] *Last's Anatomy*, 3rd edition, page 134.

[2] *Handbook of Upper Extremity Examination*: Springer, 2022, Roger Pillemer, pages 16 and 17.

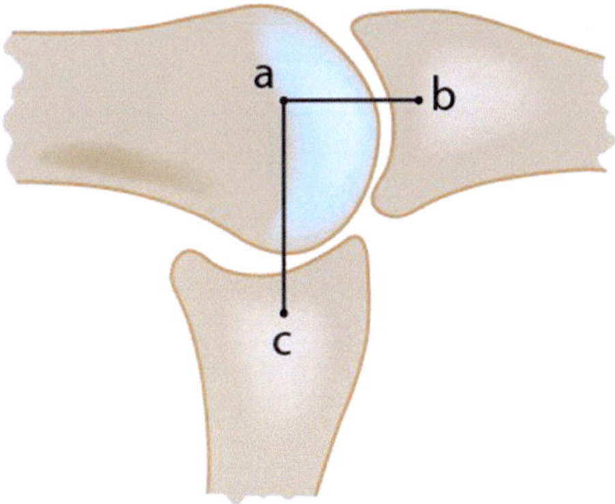

Fig. 13.5 The heads of the metacarpals are cam shaped

- These MP joints (the 'knuckle joints') lie on the arc of a circle; hence, the extended fingers diverge from each other, the flexed fingers crowd together into the palm.[3]

13.1.5 Carpometacarpal Joint of the Thumb (CMC Joint)

Verbal descriptions do not make for easy visualisation of the CMC joint of the thumb. The anatomy is best explained by noting the articular surface of the trapezium, which shows a concave articular surface dorsal to volar (red) and a convex surface radial to ulnar (blue) (Fig. 13.6). These contours are mirrored in the base of the first metacarpal (Fig. 13.7).

The shallowness of the joint provides very little stability, which is supplied by strong ligaments, both dorsal and volar. Muscles and tendons act as dynamic stabilisers.

The CMC joint allows for movements of the thumb in all three planes, with opposition being the most important movement, which allows the thumb to oppose the tip of each of the digits—precision grip.

[3]Jack Last: *Textbook of Anatomy*, 3rd edition, 1963.

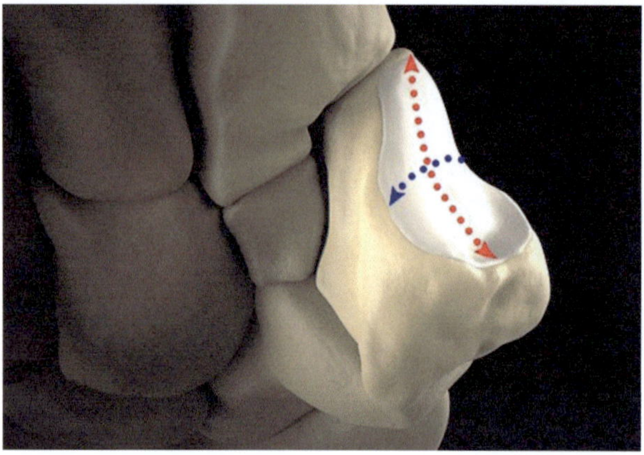

Fig. 13.6 Articular surface of trapezium

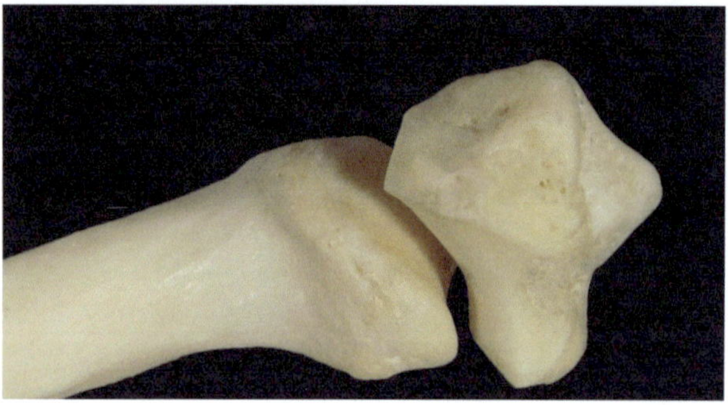

Fig. 13.7 Base of first metacarpal

13.2 Lower Extremity

13.2.1 Hip Joint

The importance of understanding the displacement in slipped capital femoral epiphysis (SCFE):[4]

[4]Pillemer R. *Handbook of Lumbar Spine and Lower Extremity Examination*: Springer, 2023, pages 92–97.

- In SCFE the epiphysis remains within the acetabulum; it is the metaphysis that slips in relation to the epiphysis.
- To be able to picture/understand the displacement that occurs, picture placing the medial side of the big toe of one foot behind the heel of the other foot (Fig. 13.8). To do this one would need to extend, adduct, and externally rotate the leg on the affected side.
- This understanding is essential in planning a corrective triplane osteotomy (Fig. 13.9).

13.2.1.1 Triplane Osteotomy

- Removal of a wedge to correct the extension and adduction deformities combined with rotation to correct the external rotation deformity (Fig. 13.9).

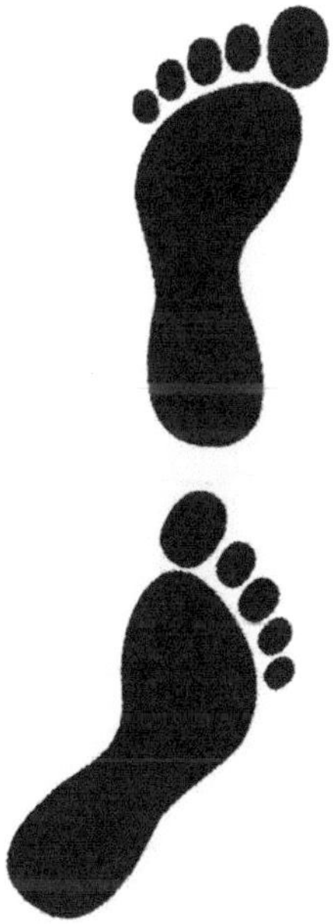

Fig. 13.8 SCFE displacement

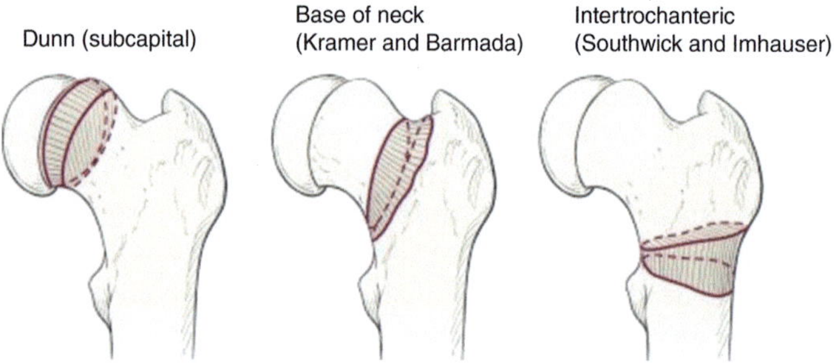

Fig. 13.9 Triplane osteotomy

13.2.2 Knee Joint

13.2.2.1 Screw Home Mechanism of the Knee

The screw home mechanism is crucial in providing knee stability.

Important Concepts

- Open chain (non-weight-bearing): The tibia is free to move, with flexion and extension movement in the sitting position. In the final stages of extension, the tibia externally rotates 10° to lock in full extension.
- Closed chain (weight-bearing): The tibia is relatively fixed, and it is the femur which moves on the tibia as in squats. In the final stages of extension, the femur internally rotates 10° to lock in full extension.

Anatomical Explanation for Locking

- The medial femoral condyle is longer than the lateral condyle, so that as full extension occurs in the open chain situation, the medial tibial condyle has slightly further to travel anteriorly, causing the 10° of external rotation.

Unlocking of the Knee

- Caused by contraction of popliteus in the open chain (Fig. 13.10).
- Caused by external rotation of the hip in closed chain.

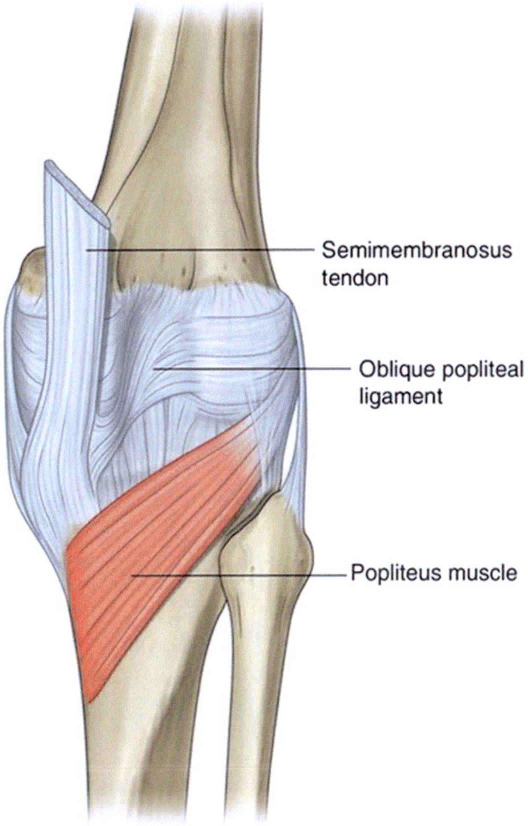

Fig. 13.10 Popliteus

In the locked position, in addition to the bony stability, the knee is held stable by tightening of all the ligaments. No muscular activity is required to maintain this stability. While standing with the knee locked, finger pressure on the patellar tendon will allow the finger to sink in (Fig. 13.11). As soon as the knee is unlocked, (starts to flex) the quadriceps contracts, the patellar tendon tightens, and the finger is 'extruded' (Fig. 13.12).

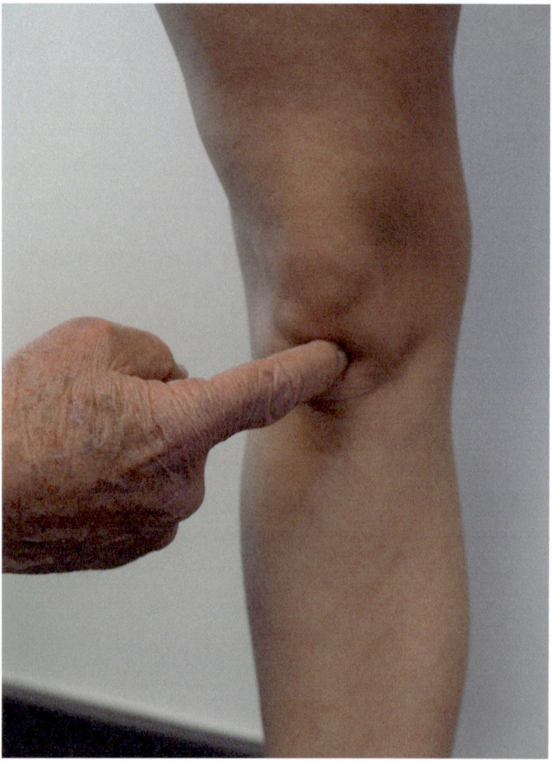

Fig. 13.11 Knee 'locked'

13.2.2.2 Summary Table

	Tibial movement	Position	Locking mechanism	Unlocking
Open chain	Mobile	Knee extension while sitting	Tibia externally rotates	Contraction of popliteus
Closed chain	Fixed	Knee extension from squatting	Femur internally rotates	External rotation of the hip

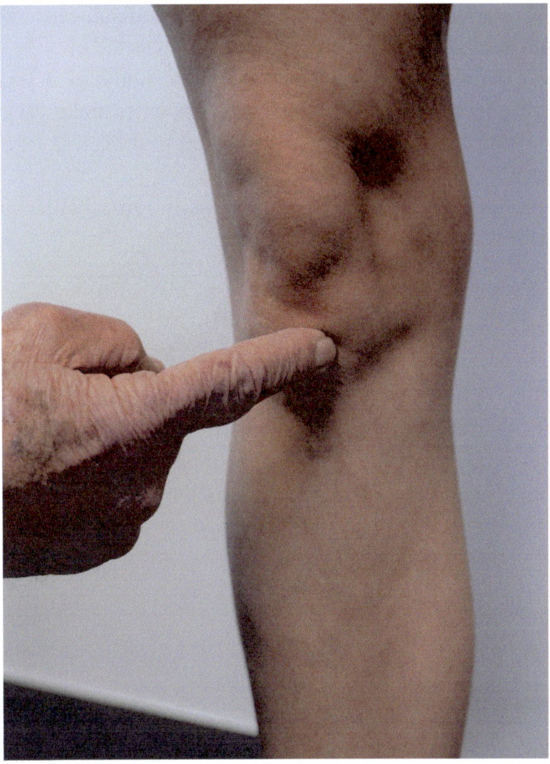

Fig. 13.12 Knee 'unlocked'

13.2.3 Ankle Joint

13.2.3.1 The Importance of Lateral Talar Shift in Ankle Fractures

An article I read in 1976 had an enormous and lasting effect on me. The authors described an in vitro experiment using a carbon black transference technique to show the reduction in the tibiotalar contact surface area associated with lateral displacement of the talus.[5] They found that with 1 mm of lateral displacement of the talus the average reduction in contact area was 42%!

These results were corroborated by a study of 12 cadaver ankles conducted in 2006[6] using carbon powder and a 70 kg load where 1 mm of lateral talar shift resulted in 40% loss of contact surface area.

These findings would seem to stress the importance of anatomical reduction in all ankle fractures.

13.2.4 Subtalar Joint

13.2.4.1 The Subtalar Joint—Measurement of Range of Movement

AMA Five describes the range of movement, and how to measure that range of movement, for every joint in the upper and lower extremities, except for inversion and eversion of the hind foot/subtalar joint (Fig. 13.13). I can suggest two possibilities for this:

(i) Simply an oversight.
(ii) No suitable method was devised.

I will suggest a remarkably simple and accurate method of assessing the range of movement of this joint, which is accurate to within one degree.

You will need to use a goniometer as illustrated (Fig. 13.14), with the fulcrum centred on the ankle joint. This happens automatically—the proximal arm of the goniometer lies against the medial aspect of the distal leg and the distal arm against the medial aspect of the calcaneus. Once you get used to using this method,

[5]Ramsey PL, Hamilton W. Changes in tibiotalar area of contact caused by lateral talar shift. *J Bone Joint Surg Am*. 1976;58(3):356–7. PMID: 1262367.

[6]Lloyd J, Elsayed S, Hariharan K, Tanaka H. Revisiting the concept of talar shift in ankle fractures. *Foot Ankle Int*. 2006;27(10):793–6. https://doi.org/10.1177/107110070602701006. PMID: 17054879.

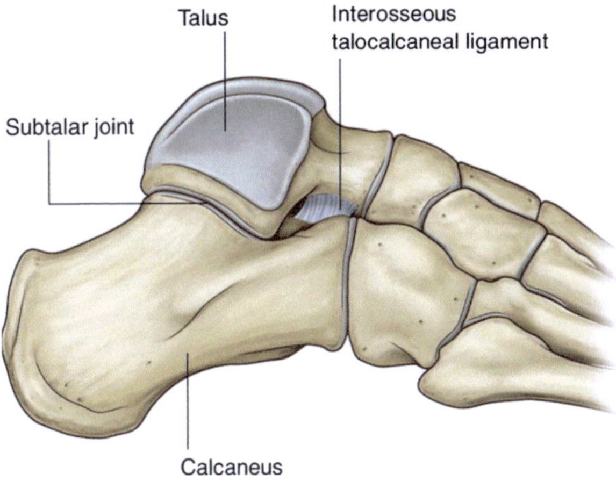

Fig. 13.13 The subtalar joint

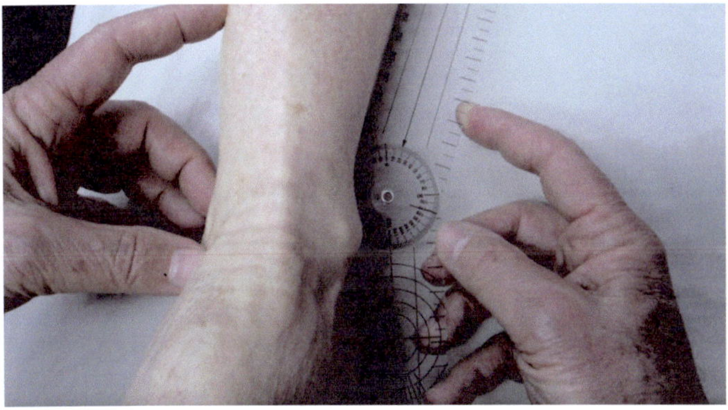

Fig. 13.14 Assessment of subtalar joint range of movement

you will see that the goniometer automatically fits into the correct position.

The starting position (Fig. 13.15) will always be in inversion because of the anatomy.

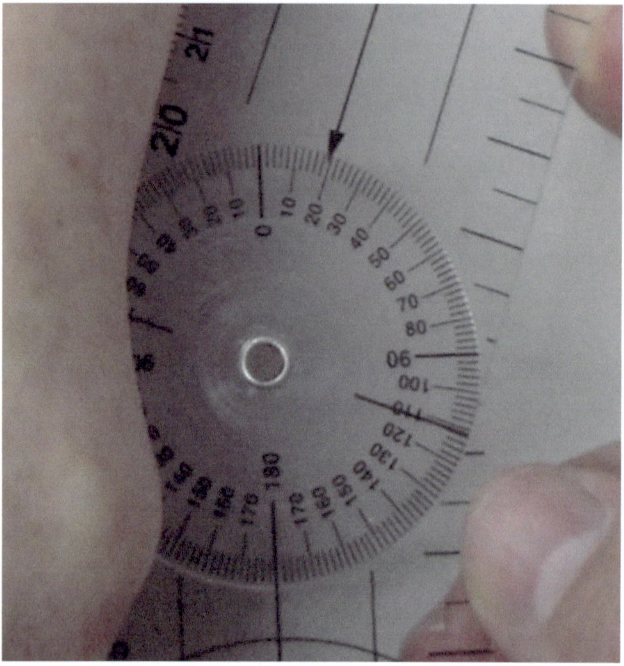

Fig. 13.15 Starting point: measurement = 20°

In this example, we measure 20°, which is our starting point. And at maximal inversion (Fig. 13.16) in this example, we measure 30°.

The actual range of inversion then is 30° − 20° = 10°.

In this example, when measuring eversion (Figs. 13.17 and 13.18), the measure was 4° giving an actual range eversion of 20° − 4° = 16°.

In summary, this method is quick, simple, and accurate. It requires three positions of the goniometer, three readings, and a bit of simple arithmetic (Fig. 13.19). Do the math and record the results.

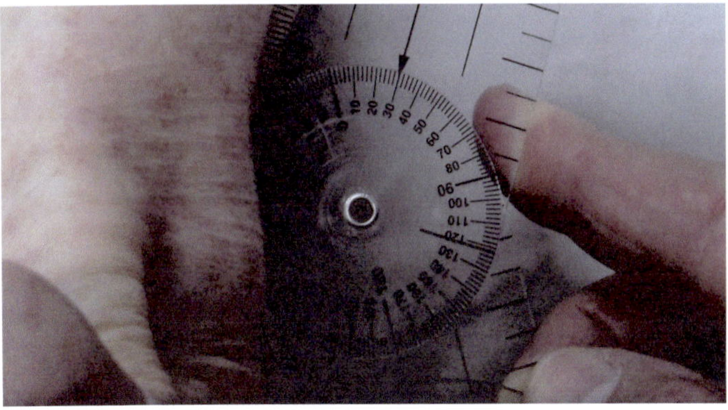

Fig. 13.16 Maximal inversion = 30°

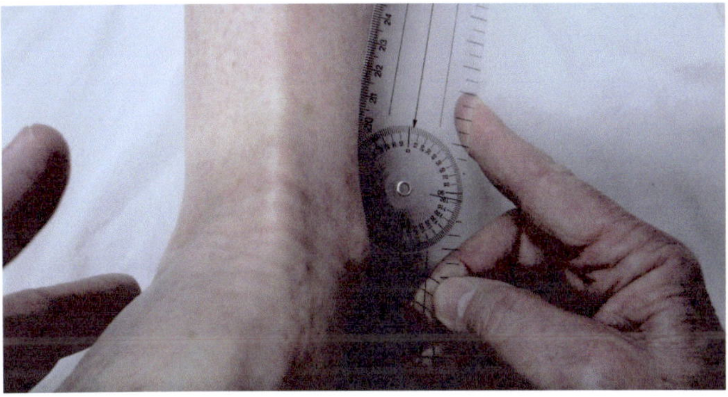

Fig. 13.17 Measuring eversion

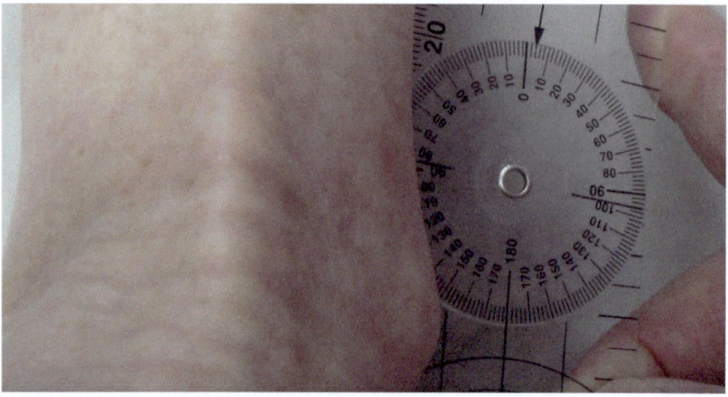

Fig. 13.18 Maximal eversion of 4°

Position of goniometer	Goniometer	Action
1	Neutral	Take a reading
2	Inversion	Take a reading
3	Eversion	Take a reading

Fig. 13.19 Goniometer positions for neutral, inversion, and eversion

Benign Bone Tumours

14

14.1 A Suggested Approach to Diagnosis

I will approach this topic under three headings:

A. The distinction between benign and malignant tumours on X-ray
B. The clinical presentation and typical findings of specific benign bone tumours on X-ray
C. A systematic approach for making a specific or differential diagnosis based on the X-ray features

With regard to signs and symptoms, tumours in relation to joints may cause pain, swelling, tenderness, and restriction of movement. In those lesions not related to joints, swelling, tenderness, or pathological fracture may be present. This section will not include discussion regarding these general non-specific features but will rather highlight the more specific details for each lesion on X-ray.

As will be noted, age is very important in determining the naturc of thc lcsion.

R. Pillemer, *Physical Signs in Orthopedic and Neurologic Disorders*, https://doi.org/10.1007/978-3-031-99529-3_14

14.1.1 The Distinction Between Benign and Malignant Tumours on X-Ray

It is generally agreed that plain X-rays are the best method of differentiating these two groups.

14.1.1.1 Malignant Tumours

Four criteria for X-ray evidence of malignancy, from the endosteum to the soft tissues (inside to out).

- Endosteal margin poorly defined (Fig. 14.1)
- Cortical erosion/destruction (Fig. 14.2)
- Periosteal reaction:
  - Sunburst effect (Fig. 14.3)
  - Elevation (Fig. 14.4)
  - Codman's triangle (Fig. 14.5)
  - Extension into soft tissues (Fig. 14.6)

14.1.1.2 Benign Tumours

In contrast to the above, benign tumours are well defined and have sclerotic borders, 'geographic'[1] bone destruction, solid periosteal reaction, and no soft tissue mass.

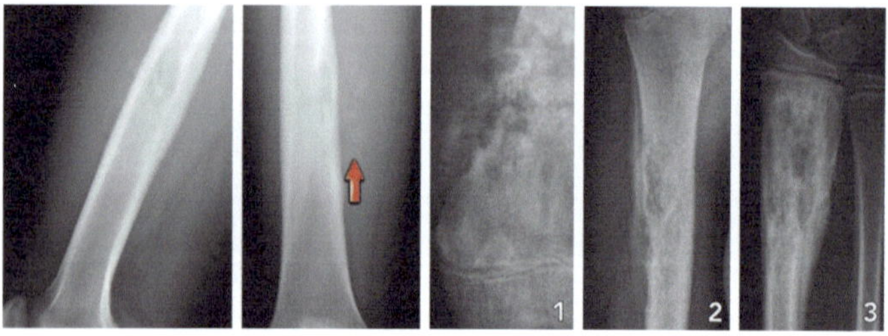

Fig. 14.1 Endosteal margin poorly defined

[1] 'Geographic' bone destruction implies a sharply defined border. The zone of transition between the lesion and the normal bone is the most important distinguishing feature between benign and malignant lesions.

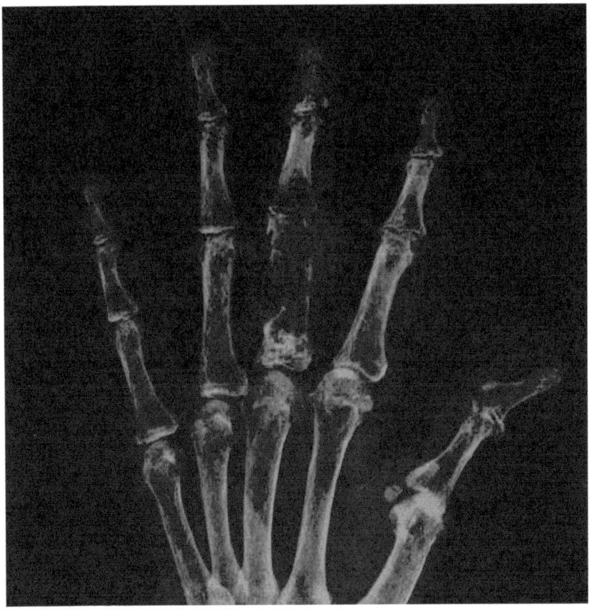

Fig. 14.2 Cortical erosion/destruction

14.1.2 The Clinical Presentation and Typical Findings of Specific Bone Tumours on X-Ray

14.1.2.1 Osteoid Osteoma

Clinical

- Age between 5 and 30
- *Pain at night improved with NSAIDS/Aspirin*
- Male to female = 3:1

X-Ray

- Figure 14.7
- 50% in proximal femur
- *Small lesion (<2 cm) with intense sclerosis surrounding radio-lucent nidus*
- Most commonly located within the cortex of the bone

Fig. 14.3 Periosteal reaction: sunburst effect

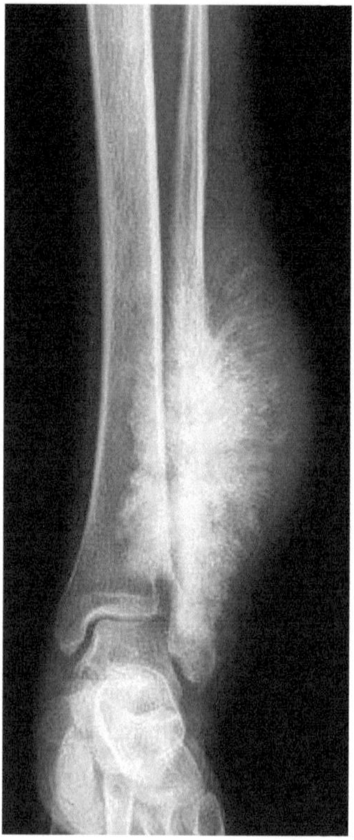

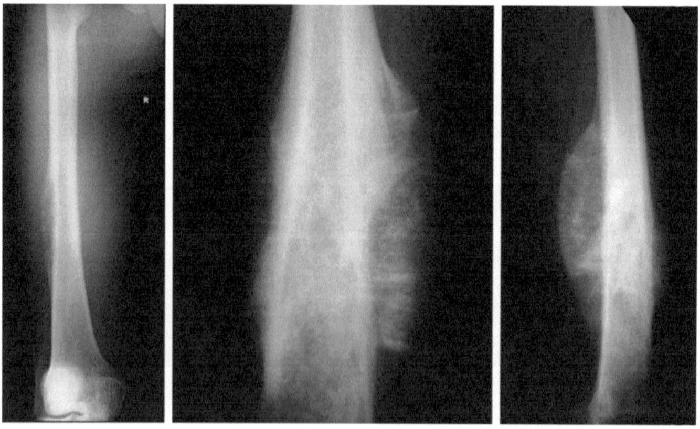

Fig. 14.4 Elevation

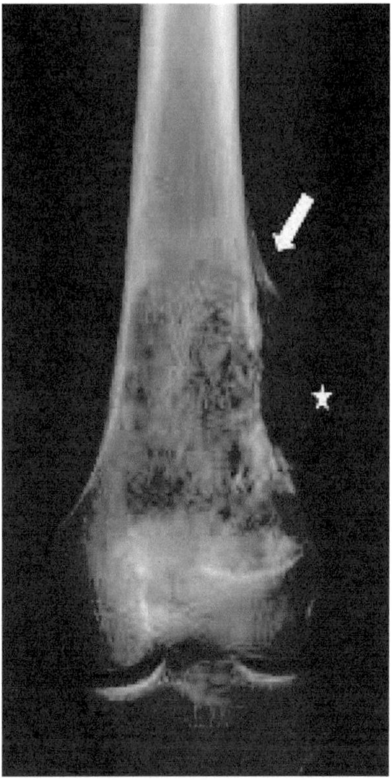

Fig. 14.5 Codman's triangle

Differential

- Osteomyelitis
- Stress fracture

14.1.2.2 Osteoblastoma

Clinical

- Age between 10 and 30; very rare; 1% of primary bone tumours
- *They differ from osteoid osteoma—in that they are found in the spine, skull and ribs. There is minimal response to NSAIDS/Aspirin*
- Male to female = 2:1

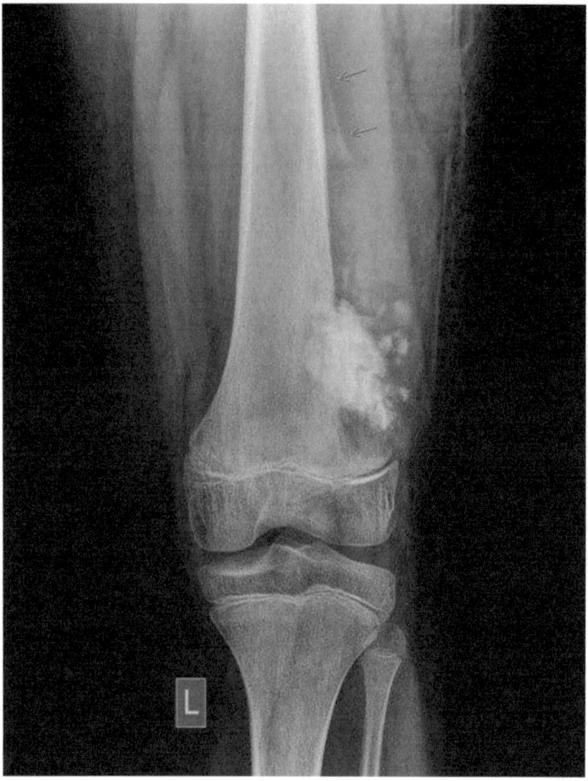

Fig. 14.6 Extension into soft tissues

X-Ray

- Figure 14.8
- Sclerotic margin with a radiolucent nidus (>2 cm)
- Most commonly found in the posterior elements of the spine
- Frequently nodular or lobulated

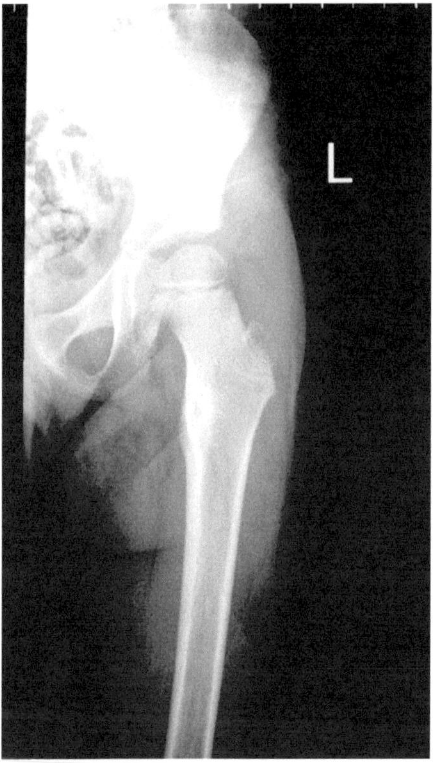

Fig. 14.7 Osteoid osteoma

Differential

- Osteoid osteoma
- Osteomyelitis
- Aneurysmal bone cyst (ABC)

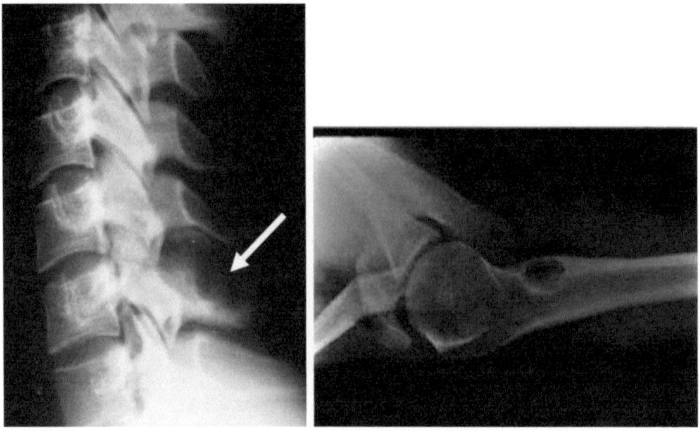

Fig. 14.8 Osteoblastoma

14.1.2.3 Giant Cell Tumour (GCT)

Clinical

- Age between 20 and 40; rare, one per million of the population
- Most commonly in the lower femur, upper tibia, or distal radius, and in the distal epiphysis commonly extending to the subchondral bone
- Slightly more common in females

X-Ray

- Figure 14.9
- Eccentric lytic lesion at the end of the long bone with a narrow transition zone as opposed to the usual sclerotic rim of other benign lesions
- There may be an expansion of the involved area

Differential

- Chondroblastoma
- Brown tumour (hyperparathyroidism) (HPT)

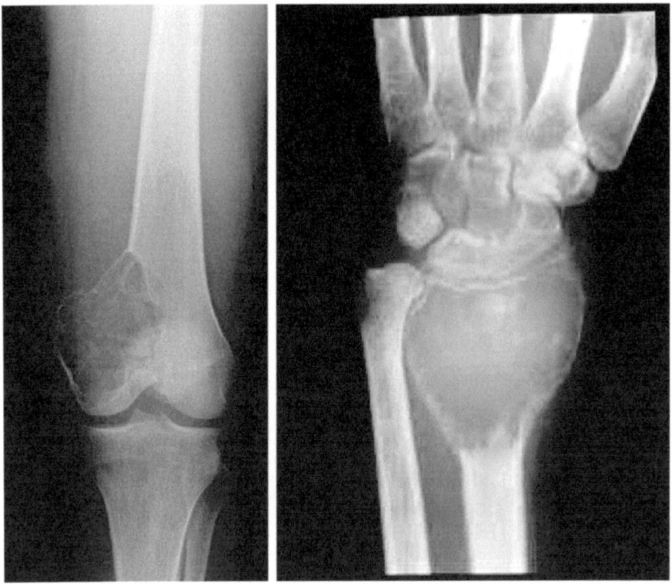

Fig. 14.9 Giant cell tumour (GCT)

14.1.2.4 Pigmented Villonodular Synovitis (PVNS)

(A tumour of synovium and not bone but can cause bone cysts due to pressure erosion, and therefore needs to be considered in the differential diagnosis.)

Clinical

- Age between 20 and 50
- Knee joint most commonly involved (80%)
- Male = female
- Can cause significant swelling

X-Ray

- Figure 14.10
- Once erosions occur, they are well defined with a sclerotic rim
- *Can involve both sides of the joint*
- No calcification

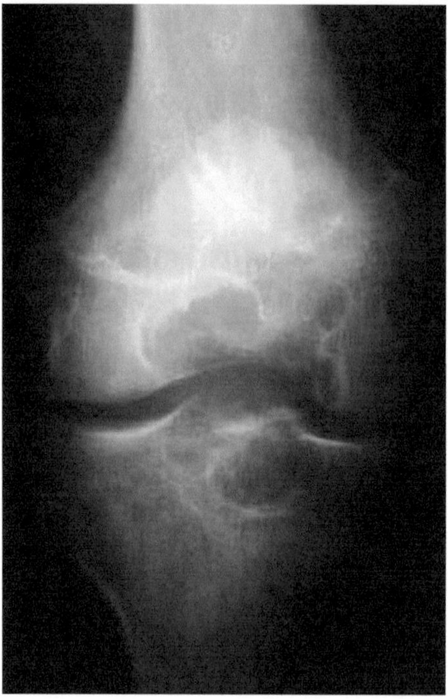

Fig. 14.10 Pigmented villonodular synovitis (PVNS)

Differential

- Gout
- Synovial chondromatosis
- Haemophilic arthropathy

14.1.2.5 Fibrous Cortical Defect (FCD)

Clinical

- Age between 5 and 15 years
- Occur in the metaphyses of long bones
- 80% in distal femur, proximal and distal tibia
- Usually asymptomatic but may present with a pathological fracture

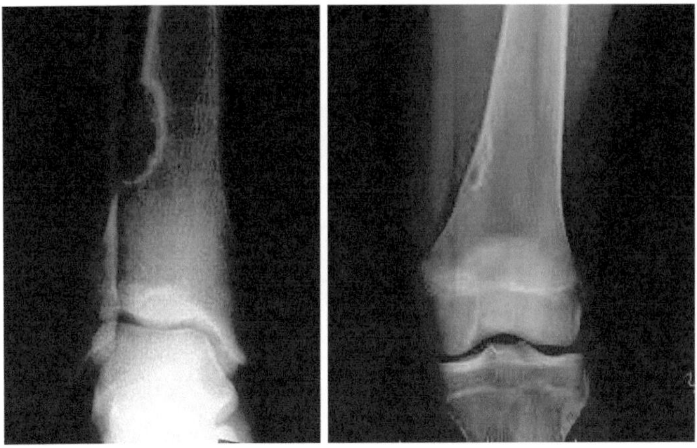

Fig. 14.11 Fibrous cortical defect (FCD)

X-Ray

- Figure 14.11
- Lucent defects within the cortex <2–3 cm
- Occur in the metaphysis or diametaphyseal junction

Differential

- Giant cell tumour
- Osteoid osteoma
- Bone abscess

14.1.2.6 Cartilage Capped Exostosis: Osteochondroma

Clinical

- The most common benign bone tumour with a cartilage cap
- Age: 10–30 years
- Painless mass
- Should not enlarge after skeletal maturity (raises concern regarding malignancy)

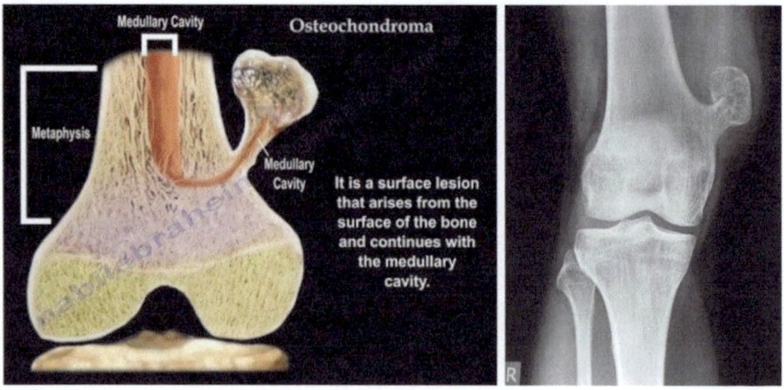

Fig. 14.12 Osteochondroma

X-Ray

- Figure 14.12
- Surface lesion in the metaphysis of long bones
- Sessile or pedunculated (if pedunculated, point away from the adjacent joint)
- Medullary and cortical continuity (the cortex and medullary cavity of the lesions are continuous with those of the host bone; this is pathognomonic)

Differential

- Subperiosteal haematoma
- Parosteal osteosarcoma
- Subungual exostosis

14.1.2.7 Enchondroma

Clinical

- Second most common benign cartilage lesion
- Most common benign hand tumour, especially in the proximal phalanx of the digits. Also occurs in large tubular bones
- Age 20–50 years; male: female = 1:1
- Asymptomatic and generally discovered incidentally unless associated with a pathological fracture

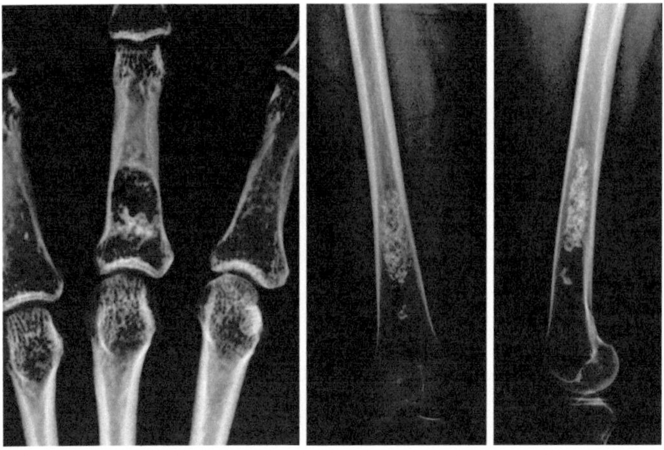

Fig. 14.13 Enchondroma

X-Ray

- Figure 14.13.
- Small (<5 cm), well-defined tumours in the middle of the bone.
- Arise in the metaphyseal region and often seen in the diaphysis.
- X-ray appearance usually includes white spots (calcification).
- May show endosteal 'scalloping' but no periosteal reaction.

Differential

- Chondrosarcoma

There are two syndromes associated with multiple enchondromas:

1. Ollier disease: (Fig. 14.14)
    - The lesions expand the bone and cause skeletal deformities.
2. Maffucci's syndrome: (Fig. 14.15)
    - As above, with cutaneous lesions composed of blood vessels.

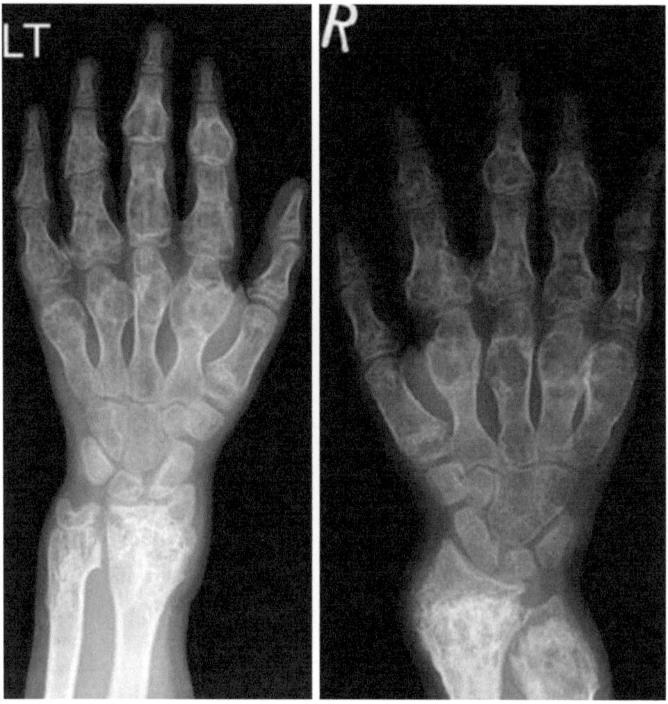

Fig. 14.14 Ollier disease: bone expansion and skeletal deformity. Ollier disease

14.1.2.8 Chondroblastoma

Clinical

- Rare, less than 1% of bone tumours
- Ages 10–20, commonest age 12 years
- Male:female = 2:1

X-Ray

- Figure 14.16.
- Well-defined eccentric lesion with sclerotic rim.
- Most commonly found in the epiphysis of the proximal tibia, distal femur, and proximal humerus.
- Lesion may cross the physis into the metaphysis.
- Stippled calcification in up to 50% of cases.

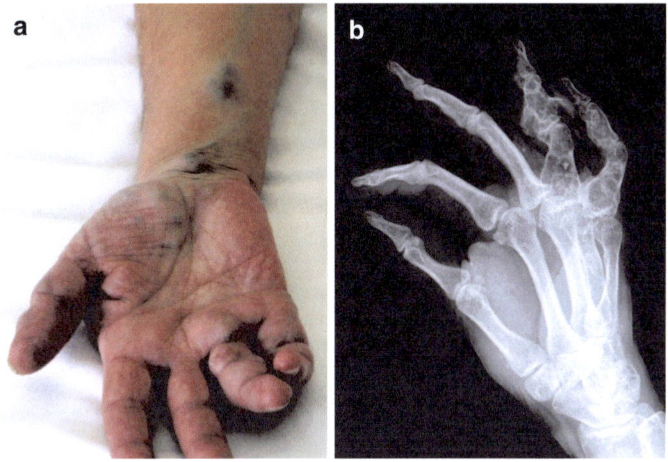

Fig. 14.15 Maffucci's syndrome (Tricò et al. *J Endocrin Soc* (2017) 1: 51–56) (a) vascular cutaneous lesions associated with (b) bone expansion and skeletal deformity

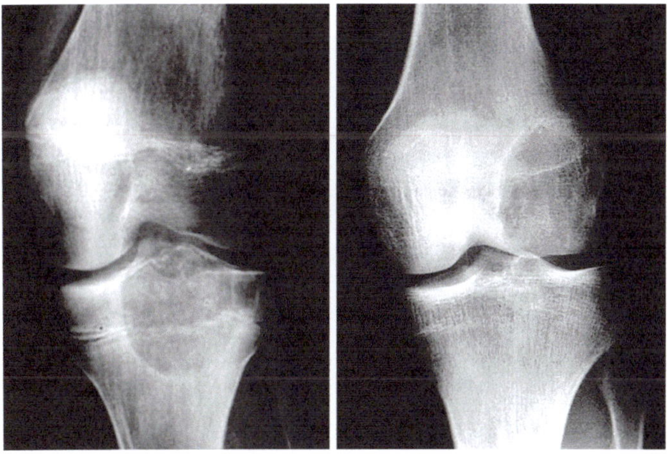

Fig. 14.16 Chondroblastoma

Differential

- Giant cell tumour
- Clear cell chondrosarcoma
- Aneurysmal bone cyst
- Osteoblastoma

14.1.2.9 Chondromyxoid Fibroma (CMF)

Clinical

- Rare (under 1%), slow growing
- Ages 10–30
- Male = female

X-Ray

- Figure 14.17.
- Eccentric metaphyseal lesion, lytic.
- Scalloped and sclerotic rim (often white); 2–6 cm.
- Sharp demarcation.
- Cortical expansion may occur.

Differential

- Aneurysmal bone cyst
- Giant cell tumour
- Central chondrosarcoma

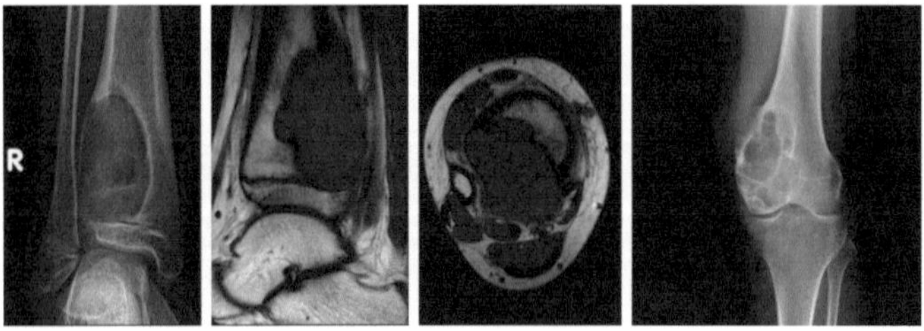

Fig. 14.17 Chondromyxoid fibroma (CMF)

14.1.2.10 Fibrous Dysplasia

Clinical

- 5% of benign bone lesions
- Monostotic: polyostotic = 4:1
- Males = females
- All age groups, usually inactive after puberty

X-Ray

- Figure 14.18
- Ribs and proximal femur >50%
- Intramedullary, expansile lesion
- Cystic, lucent, homogeneous, with endosteal scalloping and cortical thinning, no periosteal reaction
- May contain a ground-glass matrix

Differential

- Simple bone cyst
- Giant cell tumour
- Enchondromatosis

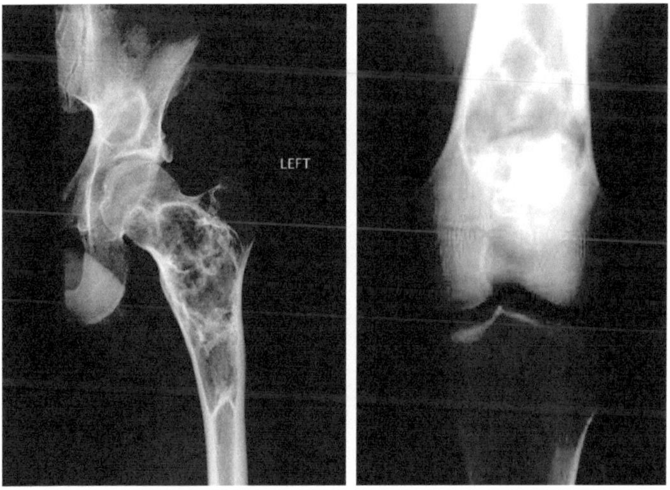

Fig. 14.18 Fibrous dysplasia

14.1.2.11 Brodie Abscess (Infection)

Clinical

- Focus of subacute/chronic pyogenic osteomyelitis
- Any location, any age

X-Ray

- Figure 14.19
- Protean features
- Predilection for metaphysis of tubular bones
- Intramedullary lesion, oval, radiolucent, well demarcated
- Surrounding sclerosis and cortical thickening
- Periosteal reaction

Differential

- Osteoid osteoma
- Eosinophilic granuloma
- Sarcoma

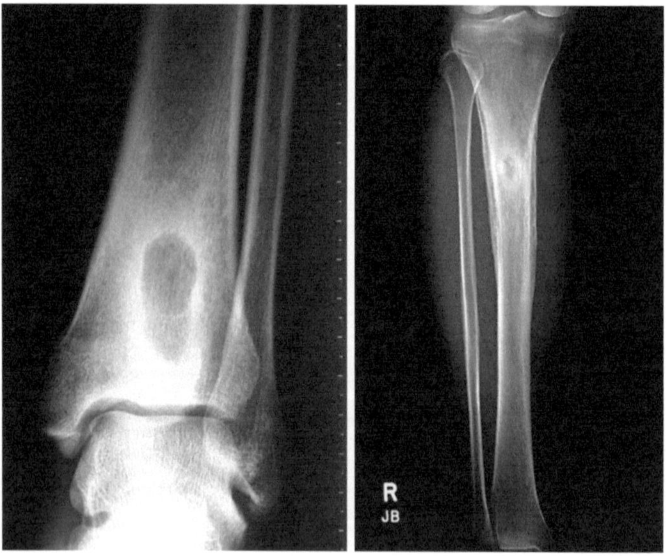

Fig. 14.19 Brodie abscess (infection)

14.1.2.12 Aneurysmal Bone Cyst (ABC)

Clinical

- Uncommon lesions
- Most commonly presents under 20 years of age
- Commonest sites around the knee
- May present with swelling or palpable mass

X-Ray

- Figure 14.20
- Radiolucent cystic lesion in metaphysis
- May expand cortical bone with thin shell of cortex
- Usually eccentric
- Bony septae; 'bubbly appearance'

Differential

- Giant cell tumour
- Chondromyxoid fibroma
- Chondroblastoma
- Simple bone cyst
- Fibrous dysplasia

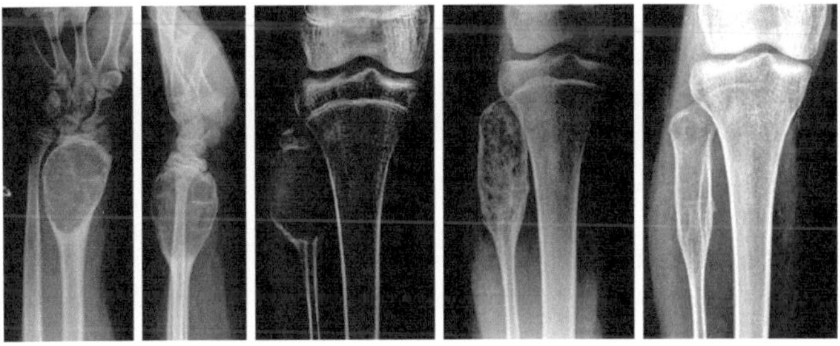

Fig. 14.20 Aneurysmal bone cyst (ABC)

14.1.2.13 Simple (Unicameral) Bone Cyst

Clinical

- Ages 5–15 years
- 3% of bone tumours
- Males: females = 2:1
- 90% occur in proximal humerus or proximal femur
- Rare in adults—suggests spontaneous resolution

X-Ray

- Figure 14.21
- Central, lytic, fluid-filled, well demarcated metaphyseal lesion; migrates to diaphysis with bone growth
- Thinning of cortices, may present with pathological fracture
- 'Fallen leaf'[2] sign—pathognomonic

Differential

- Aneurysmal bone cyst
- Enchondroma
- Fibrous dysplasia
- GCT
- Eosinophilic granuloma

14.1.2.14 Hyperparathyroidism: Brown Tumour

- Form of osteitis fibrosa cystica (OFC)—any cause of excess osteoclastic activity

Clinical

- Rare lesion
- Women: men = 5:4—5th to 6th decade
- Can affect any bone but most common in maxilla and mandible, ribs, clavicle, pelvis
- Can expand the shape of the bone and cause bone pain
- May have features of hyperparathyroidism

[2] 'Fallen leaf sign': Following pathological fracture, a bony fragment may sink to the bottom of the cyst.

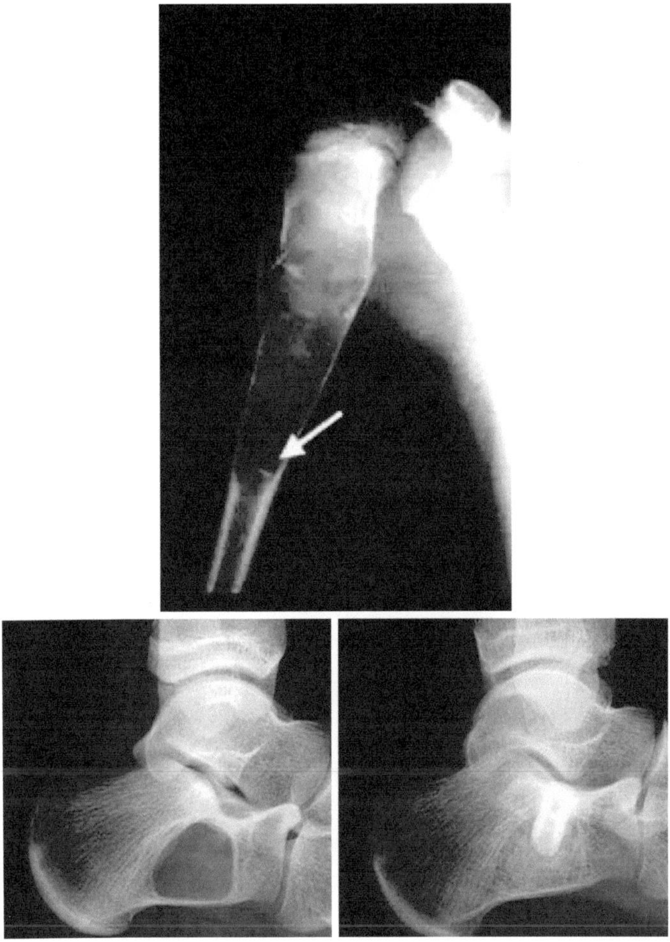

Fig. 14.21 Simple (unicameral) bone cyst

X-Ray

- Figure 14.22
- Simple or multiple well defined osteolytic lesions
- Radiolucent, subperiosteal resorption and osteopenia
- Bone expansion—pathological fractures
- Can be ill-defined with mixed lytic/sclerotic lesion or margin
- Can be soft tissue involvement

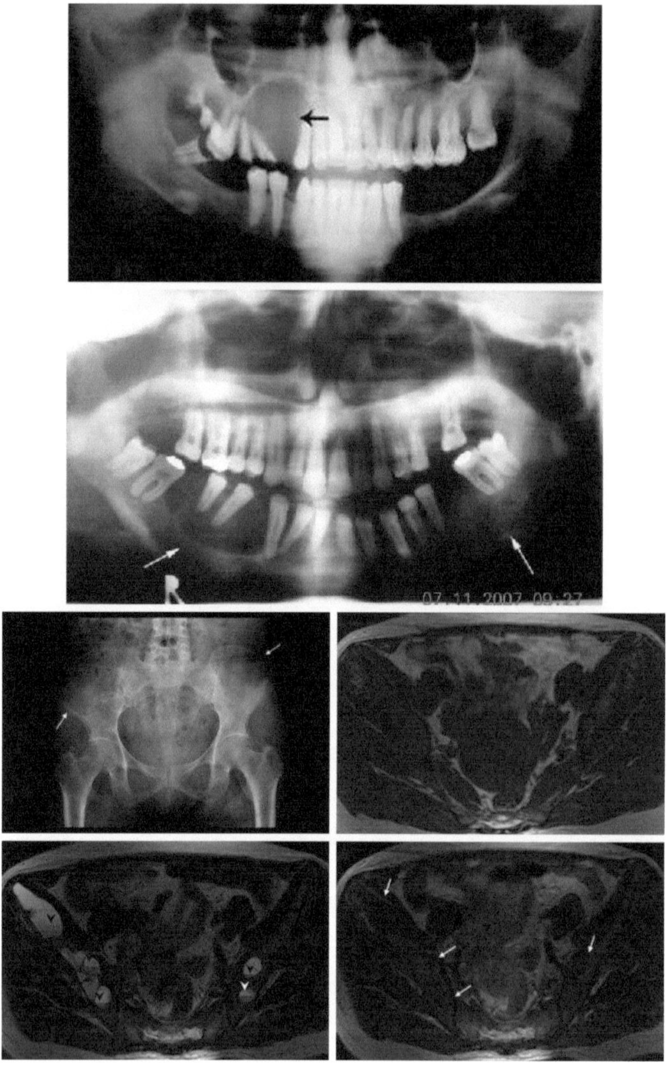

Fig. 14.22 Hyperparathyroidism (Brown tumour)

Differential

- Giant cell tumour
- Aneurysmal bone cyst
- Metastases/multiple myeloma—consider in any case with multifocal osteolytic bone lesions

14.1.2.15 Histiocytosis X: Eosinophilic Granuloma (EG)

- EG is the mildest form of Langerhans cell histiocytosis, the other two forms being Hand-Schuller-Christian disease and Letterer-Siwe disease

Clinical

- Benign self-limiting lesions which can spontaneously resolve
- Most common in children 4–10 years old and up to 4th decade
- Males: females = 2:1
- Common sites are the skull (in children), thoracic spine, ribs, clavicle, scapula
- May have pain and swelling at site

X-Ray

- Figure 14.23.
- Referred to as 'The great mimicker'.
- Cranial: multiple 'punched out' lytic lesions.
- Spinal: flattened vertebra (vertebra plana).
- Diaphyseal: intramedullary 'punched out' lesions.
- Cortical lesions could result in the cortex being thinned, expanded or destroyed. There may be periosteal involvement.
- Metaphyseal: lesions may extend to the physis but not through it.

Differential

- Osteomyelitis
- Ewing's sarcoma
- Fibrous dysplasia
- Enchondroma
- Leukaemia

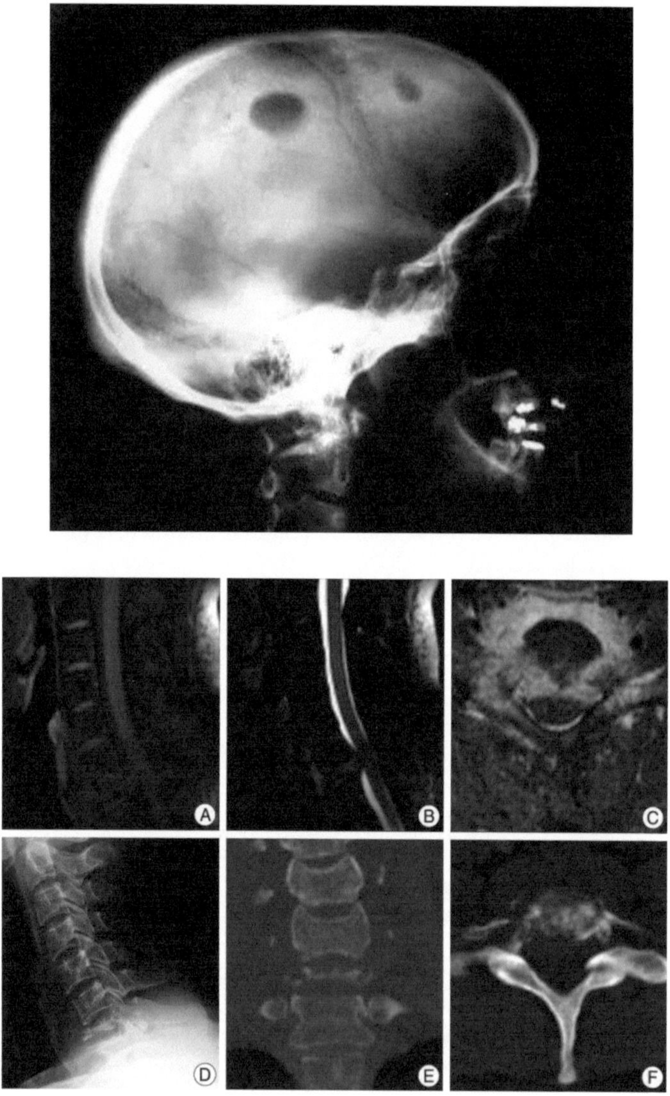

Fig. 14.23 Histiocytosis X: Eosinophilic granuloma (EG)

14.1.3 A Systematic Approach to Making a Specific/Differential Diagnosis When Presented with an X-Ray of a Benign Bone Tumour

Unless one deals with bone tumours on a regular basis, making a diagnosis of a benign bone tumour on x-ray can be very confusing and confronting. It is often difficult to suggest a diagnosis or differential diagnosis without a well-planned familiar system.

In Sect. 14.1.2, I have indicated the characteristic features of each of these lesions.

In order to consider each possible diagnosis, a routine order is suggested. A 'tick' is given to any lesion that could fit the picture and could therefore be included in the differential diagnosis.

If you practice this method, a few times you will be fairly confident of noting all of the possibilities in any particular case.

My suggestion is that you use the mnemonic: '*2 3 4 FLASH*'

The *2* represents the two bony lesions:

- Osteoid osteoma
- Osteoblastoma

The *3* refers to the three lesions represented by acronyms:

- GCT—Giant cell tumour
- PVNS—Pigmented villonodular synovitis
- FCD—Fibrous cortical defect

The *4* represents the four chondral lesions:

- Cartilage capped exostosis (Osteochondroma)
- Enchondroma
- Chondroblastoma
- Chondromyxoid fibroma

The FLASH represents:

F: Fibrous dysplasia.
L: Represents spiroketal (*L*ues) and bacterial infection. That is, a Brodie's abscess.
A: Aneurysmal bone cyst.
S: Simple bone cyst.
H: Histiocytosis 'X' → Eosinophilic granuloma
Hyperparathyroidism → Brown tumours.

15 Tips and Timesavers in Medicolegal Reporting

Most of the English-speaking countries of the world, as well as many countries in Europe, Hong Kong, and the Middle East, use the American Medical Association Guides, editions four, five, and six, in the assessment of impairment. In all jurisdictions, the final assessment will be influenced by the prevailing legal system.

The aim of this chapter is not a guide of how to draft a medicolegal report, but to share with you my thoughts on 'tips and timesavers' that I have used over many years of doing medicolegal assessments.

The topics will be discussed under the following headings:

- Dealing with the paperwork
- Preparation of the file
- The consultation
- The 'golden rule'
- The report
- Macros
- Biased reporting
- Tables and laminates

To avoid repetition, I will leave out the words 'In my opinion…' in relation to statements made. All statements are to be prefaced in this way.

R. Pillemer, *Physical Signs in Orthopedic and Neurologic Disorders*, https://doi.org/10.1007/978-3-031-99529-3_15

While certainly accepting that we all have our own way of doing medicolegal reports and noting that many of my suggestions will not suit your own style, I am extremely optimistic that by the end of the chapter, you will have found something that will save you time in the future.

As a guarantee of this, let me refer you to page 235 headed 'Range of Motion Table'. Using this table will make reading this whole chapter worthwhile, and in fact the whole book worthwhile, if you engage in doing medicolegal reports. This page is brilliant and was suggested by my friend and colleague Dr Brian Noll. If you use this table, you will never have to use a Pie Chart ever again! This page will save you many hours and much effort in the future. I suggest that you enlarge the page, print it out, and laminate it, and I guarantee that you will never leave home without it!

Very importantly, you need to leave sufficient time for the consultation, and for musculoskeletal assessments, this needs to be a minimum of 1 h (see Sect. 15.4).

15.1 Dealing with the Paperwork

One is often faced with hundreds of pages of documents, many of which are critical, such as medical reports, and others of doubtful value. Simply sorting these documents, which require no special medical or legal knowledge, can take a considerable time.

I, therefore, have an assistant, usually a university student, who will go through the paperwork for me, sorting and tagging all medical reports, investigations, patient statements, and any other relevant documents. I pay her twice as much as she would receive pulling beers in a pub at night, and everyone is happy!

In addition, and most importantly, my assistant will also list *factual information* such as:

- Dates of each operation, the procedure carried out, and the name of the treating specialist
- Any other forms of treatment that the patient may have had
- Present treatment
- Details of the work history

Please note that all the information noted above is *factual information*. The significance and importance of this will be discussed under the Sect. 15.3.

General practitioner and other contemporaneous reports such as ambulance and hospital reports are also collated. These may be important regarding pre-existing condition, severity of the injury, body parts involved, immediate post-injury treatment, and response to same. Injured workers' memories are often hazy about these facts, and contemporaneous reports can be immensely helpful.

15.2 Preparation of the File

The key to a good medicolegal report is in the preparation of the file. Once the documentation has been sorted, and if one is dealing with a straight-forward case, say an amputation of a digit, then obviously minimal time needs to be spent on the preparation of the file.

However, in complex cases where multiple body parts may be involved, and where causation needs to be considered, an appropriate time needs to be devoted, so that by the time of the consultation, you will have a clear understanding of:

- What the critical issues are.
- What specific questions need to be asked.
- What specific signs need to be looked for.

15.3 The Consultation Process

As noted, prior to the consultation you will have listed all the factual information. The reason that this is so important is that this information then needs to be CONFIRMED and not ELICITED. Imagine the man who has had a nailing for a tibial fracture that has gone on to non-union and requires a revision procedure with bone grafting and a final operation to remove prominent screws. It might take you 10 min to try and elicit this information compared to 5 s to simply confirm, e.g. 'Jack, I note that you have had three operations on your leg, the last being about a year ago'.

Similarly, getting a work history form the patient since the injury 4 years previously, with the varying periods of time off, time on selective duties, present situation, may take another 10 min. Compare this to your prepared notes: 'I note that you had 6 months off after the original injury, and further time off after each of your operations. You have always been back on selective duties and on reduced hours, but that in the last 8 months you have been back full time but only in the warehouse and not in the field'. Another 10 min saved.

You have now saved 20 min which can be devoted to a detailed history of current symptoms and a careful physical examination. I repeat, *factual information only needs to be confirmed not elicited.* This will obviously not apply when say causation is in doubt, when much time may be needed to get an accurate history.

You also need to decide how much time to leave for the consultation plus the time needed to dictate your report (see Sect. 15.4). This needs to be a minimum of 1 h, which takes into account the time saved by confirming factual information.

The majority of patients are very anxious as the consultation is often critical for their futures. They may have been waiting a long time to get the appointment and very often have seen specialists who they feel have treated them badly, either by rushing them through the consultation and not giving them time to answer the questions, or who have been rude and they felt that they were talked down to.

It is important then to try and get the patient to relax, particularly if you are seeing them for the insurance company. You will already be regarded as 'the insurance company doctor' and/or 'on the other side'. There are a number of ways to do this:

- A friendly/smiling welcome with a handshake if appropriate.
- I address the person by their first name and introduce myself by my first name, again if appropriate, and welcome any companion in the same way.

- Start by asking some broad questions, for example, if the patient has a suitcase, ask where they have come from.
- I thank them for being early/on time.
- If they have an accent and/or are obviously not 'locals' I ask where they were from originally. And I certainly do not regard this as racist, although these days many suggest that it might be.
- If I am seeing say a 75-year-old female, I might say 'It says here that you are 75—that can't be right'. You will be miles ahead in getting the patient to relax.
- I point out the prepared files with all the stickers and tell the patient that I have been through all the notes, and I know what is going on, so that he/she will have plenty of time to tell me everything they think I need to know.
- It is essential that the patient does not feel rushed or 'spoken down to', as this is not fair to the patient nor to our profession.

I am always pleased when the wife/partner also attends, as in general males tend to be hopeless with dates. I may say for example: 'Jack I note that you had a radical prostatectomy—when was that?' They generally have no idea and tend to either look blank, shrug their shoulders, supinate the hands as though catching two tennis balls, turn pleadingly to the wife, or all the above. The wife will then say something like 'It was on the 10th of June 2019, the week after Helen's wedding'. Females tend to relate events to each other. Males tend to be oblivious.

The key point in mentioning this, and as discussed in the preparation of the file, trying to elicit the dates and details of previous operations is frustrating and time consuming. *It is factual information. It is CONFIRMED and not ELICITED.* What might have taken you 10 min, now takes a few seconds.

This will leave you with extra time for the important aspects of the consultation, namely, a detailed history of present symptoms and time to conduct an unrushed examination. How often does the patient tell you that the last doctor spent less than 10 min on the consultation.

Regarding investigations, I always view these in front of the patient, mainly for my own education and edification. Very often the patient will then say that I am the only doctor who has looked at the x-rays.

At the end of the consultation, I say something like: 'Sam, I have all the information I need. Is there anything else you think that I need to know about that we have not discussed'. I then sit back in my chair as if I have all the time in the world and let Sam talk. Occasionally there may be some additional relevant information, but it is really only a time to let the patient gets things off their chest, such as how poorly he has been treated by his employer whom he has worked for, for over 15 years, how the insurance company has tried to cut him off at every turn, how his whole life has changed and his partner has left the relationship, etc.

The patients usually run out of things to say after a couple of minutes. It is particularly important to allow the patient to feel that they have been heard.

15.4 The 'Golden Rule'

If you take nothing else from this chapter, let it be this.

As soon as the patient leaves the consulting room, I close the door and do the dictation there and then. The staff know that I am not to be disturbed at this time.

There are so many reasons for this:

- Everything is fresh in my mind.
- I do not have to write copious notes, which I would have to do if I were to dictate at a later stage.
- There is no confusion with other cases seem on the same day as must occur with delayed dictation, particularly if the delay is more that say a few hours.
- I again have no doubt that what would take 20 min of dictation time when carried out immediately would take at least twice as long if carried out 24 h later, with a progressive increase in time taken the longer the delay.

- When dictation is delayed to that night, or later, instead of having to try and think back to the examination, and anxiously try to recall whether the calf wasting was on the right or left side, I can, in a more relaxed fashion, start preparing the files for the following week. A much more effective, and efficient use of the same amount of time.

I am always bemused when I see a medical report where the examination was carried out on say the first of the month, but the date of the report is the tenth of the month or later. I can only imagine the number of pages of written notes that would have been needed to enable dictation 10 days later.

The added advantage of immediate dictation is that my typist is able to start typing the report straight away and I will get the draft back within 2 h. I can then do the corrections and the paperwork can be lodged on the day of the consultation, or certainly within 24 h. This can only happen if both you and your typist are up to date. Being up to date also allows for supplementary reports to be answered on the same day.

If you are not already using the Golden Rule, please try it. As noted at the outset, it is most important to leave sufficient time for the consultation that also allows for the time needed for the dictation.

To repeat, if you only take one suggestion from this chapter, let it be Sect. 15.4.

15.5 The Report

It is helpful to start your report with a summary of your conclusions so that the reader knows what the key issues are and the direction in which you are heading.

Many non-medical people will be reading your report, and it is therefore important to use writing that is easy to understand and avoids non-medical terms. Where medical terms are used, an explanation should be given, for example: 'Mr Jones has a positive Tinel's sign, that is, tapping over the carpal tunnel produces parasthesias that radiate into the median nerve supplied digits'.

Avoid the use of Latin/non-English phrases in your report.

Where possible use tables to show the range of movement with the associated impairment rather than having this information simply in a paragraph. This makes it so much easier for anyone checking your report to confirm the figures of impairment.

There is a tendency to 'pad' reports to make them seem longer and more substantial. Be as succinct as possible. I am reminded of the phrase: 'Perfection is finally attained, not when there is no longer anything to add, but when there is no longer anything to take away'.

15.6 Macros

Dictation macros are used to substitute frequently used text and references, by having a code of which both you and your typist have a copy.

Many non-medical people will need to check your reports and in order to do so will need to use the references in your reports to the various tables and figures in the AMA Guides.

It is helpful, and in some jurisdictions required, that these references be given. For example, if you have made the statement that 'Mr Jones falls into DRE Category lll of his lumber spine (1) with 10% WPI', in the appropriate section you will list (1) as follows:

AMA Guides to the Evaluation of Permanent Impairment Fifth Edition:

(1) Page 384, Table 15-3. Significant signs of radiculopathy.

Or 'Mr Jones has restriction of left shoulder movement as noted in the attached worksheet which entitles him to 12% upper extremity impairment' (2)

This would then read:

(2) Page 476 Fig. 16-40, page 477 Fig. 16-43, page 479 Fig. 16-46.

Using macros will save you and your typist an enormous amount of time and will be greatly appreciated by the typist!

15.7 Biased Reporting

As the man once said, 'We are all biased'.

Discussion of bias requires a whole chapter on its own but needs to be mentioned, so I will simply highlight a few prominent issues.

Let me start by suggesting that there are two kinds of bias, 'Intrinsic' and 'Extrinsic'. Intrinsic bias is very personal and an example of this type of bias is seen when two lawyers in a TV show discuss an upcoming trial, one says 'I hope that we do not get Judge X; you know what he will decide'.

Extrinsic bias occurs when your reports are favourable to the referrer, and there are obvious reasons for this, including financial, social, 'wanting to please'. Solicitors from either side will tell you that they want your genuine opinion, but this is usually not the case, and they would prefer a report that favours their client. We all have a tendency to be biased, and it is something that one has to actively work against.

You might not be aware of, or thought of, the fact that all of your medical colleagues who read your reports, as well as case managers, solicitors, barristers, and even judges, have a fair idea of where your bias lies. Despite this, it is not unusual for the doctor not to be aware that they are writing biased reports, and this can be conscious or unconscious.

The first step then is to determine whether one is writing biased reports. Might I tactfully suggest that if you are only writing reports for the worker's solicitors, or alternatively for the insurance company or their representatives, it is highly likely that you are writing biased reports.

After acknowledgement of this, the second step is to have a method to try and prevent it. My suggestion is that once you have completed your report, ask yourself 'If I had been doing this report for the other side, would it have been any different?' If the answer is 'Yes', then go back and change what needs to be changed, even if this is only a nuance.

Please note that this is not a rhetorical or theoretical question, but a question one literally needs to ask oneself at the completion of every report.

We are all aware of our colleagues who are known and respected for their unbiased reports. Aim to be one of this group!

15.8 Tables and Laminates

Please find attached five tables which I have laminated and have with me at all times when doing impairment assessments (printed front and back, three laminated pages in total).

- Range of motion table, which I referred to above, is the most useful, single time-saving page ever.
- Range of motion work sheets which both my typist and I have, so that when I dictate the figures for range of movement, I only have to give the figures without having to indicate the direction of movement.
- Index Table: This shows the pages as well as the table/figure numbers of all the tables and figures for the upper and lower extremities as well as the lumbar spine, in both AMA4 and AMA5.
- How to convert finger/thumb impairment to hand impairment to upper extremity impairment to whole person impairment, all on one page.
- Combination tables, which we use constantly.

I hope that you will find this chapter useful in saving you time and frustration in your medicolegal reporting. If you have any further tips and timesavers to add to the above, I would be delighted to hear from you, and if there happens to be a second edition, more than happy to include your suggestions!

RANGE OF MOTION – UPPER EXTREMITIES

SHOULDER IMPAIRMENT

	0	10	20	30	40	50	60	70	80	90	100	110	120	130	140	150	160	170	180
Flex	21	16	11	10	10	9	8	7	7	6	5	5	4	3	3	2	1	1	0
Ext	3	2	2	1	1	0													
Add	2	1	1	1	0	0													
Abd	12	10	7	7	6	6	6	5	5	4	4	3	3	2	2	1	1	0	0
IR	5	5	4	4	3	2	2	1	0	0									
ER	2	2	1	1	1	1	0	0	0	0									

ELBOW IMPAIRMENT

	0	10	20	30	40	50	60	70	80	90	100	110	120	130	140
Flexion	42	37	34	31	27	23	19	15	10	8	6	4	2	1	0
Extension	0	1	2	3	4	5	6	8	11	17	21	27	32	37	42

	-80	-70	-60	-50	-40	-30	-20	-10	0	10	20	30	40	50	60	70	80
Pronation	28	27	25	24	22	21	19	15	12	8	4	3	3	2	1	1	0
Supination	28	22	18	13	8	6	4	4	3	3	3	2	2	1	1	0	0

WRIST IMPAIRMENT

	-60	-50	-40	-30	-20	-10	0	10	20	30	40	50	60
Extension	42	36	30	24	18	13	11	8	7	5	4	2	0
Flexion	42	36	25	21	17	13	10	8	7	5	3	2	0

	-30	-25	-20	-15	-10	-5	0	5	10	15	20	25	30
Radial Deviation	18	15	12	9	5	5	4	3	2	1	0		
Ulnar Deviation			18	15	12	9	5	4	4	3	2	1	0

FINGER IMPAIRMENT

		+30	+20	+10	0	10	20	30	40	50	60	70	80	90	100
MP	**Flexion**		60	54	49	44	38	33	27	22	17	11	6	0	
	Extension		0	3	5	7	10	12	27	41	56	71	85	100	
PIP	**Flexion**	80	73	66	60	54	48	42	36	30	24	18	12	6	0
	Extension	0	0	0	0	3	7	11	14	25	36	47	58	69	80
DIP	**Flexion**	45	42	39	36	31	26	21	15	10	5	0			
	Extension	0	0	0	0	2	4	12	20	29	37	45			

THUMB IMPAIRMENT

		+40	+30	+20	+10	0	10	20	30	40	50	60	70	80
MP	**Flexion**	10	9	8	7	6	5	4	3	2	1	0		
	Extension	0	0	0	0	0	1	1	3	5	8	10		
IP	**Flexion**		15	13	11	8	6	4	4	3	2	1	1	0
	Extension		0	0	0	1	2	3	5	7	9	11	13	15

	15	20	25	30	35	40	45	50
Lack of Radial Abduction	10	9	7	5	3	2	0	0
Lack of Radial Adduction	0	1	1	1	3	5	8	9

cms	0	1	2	3	4	5	6	7	8
Lack of adduction	0	0	1	3	4	6	8	13	20
Lack of opposition	45	31	22	13	9	5	3	1	0

RANGE OF MOVEMENT

UPPER EXTREMITY:

Finger		**Index**	**Middle**	**Ring**	**Little**
DIP	Flexion				
	Extension				
PIP	Flexion				
	Extension				
MP	Flexion				
	Extension				

Thumb	**Flexion**	**Extension**
MP		
IP		
Radial Abduction		
Opposition	cm	
Adduction	cm	

Wrist	**Right**	**Left**
Flexion		
Extension		
Radial Deviation		
Ulnar Deviation		

Elbow	**Right**	**Left**
Flexion		
Extension		
Pronation		
Supination		

Shoulder	**Right**	**Left**
Flexion		
Extension		
Abduction		
Adduction		
Internal rotation		
External rotation		

****

LOWER EXTREMITY:

Hip	**Right**	**Left**
Flexion		
Extension		
Internal rotation		
External rotation		
Abduction		
Adduction		

Knee	**Right**	**Left**
Flexion		
Flexion Contracture		

Ankle	**Right**	**Left**
Plantar Flexion		
Flexion Contracture		
Extension		

Hindfoot	**Right**	**Left**
Inversion		
Eversion		

Toes	**Right**	**Left**
Great Toe: MP Extension		
IP Extension		
Lesser Toes: MP Extension		

TABLE REFERENCES

AMA 4		UPPER LIMB	AMA 5	
18 f2		**Amputation:Upp. Extremity**	441 f16-2	
18 f3		**Hand**	442 f 16-3	
22 f5		**Sensory Loss Hand**	449 f 16-8	
24 f7		**Thumb: Amp/Sensory Loss**	443 f 16-4	447 f 16-6
30 f17		**Finger: Amp/Sensory Loss**	443 f 16-5	447 f 16-7
26 f10	27 f13	**Thumb**	456 f 16-12	457 f 16-15
28 t5 & 6	29 t7		459 t 16-8 a & b	460 t 16-9
32 f19	33 f21	**Finger**	461 f 16-21	463 f 16-23
34 f23			464 f 16-25	
36 f26	38 f29	**Wrist**	467 f 16-28	469 f 16-31
40 f32	41 f35	**Elbow**	472 f 16-34	474 f 16-37
43 f38	44 f41	**Shoulder**	476 f 16-40	477 f 16-43
45 f44			479 f 16-46	
48 t11(s)	49 t12(m)	**Nerve Deficits**	482 t 16-10 (s)	484 f 16-11(m)
54 t15			492 t 16-15	
57 t16		**Entrapment Neuropathy**	493	
		CRPS	496 t 16-16	
61 t27		**Arthroplasty**	506 t 16-27	
59-63		**Other**	501-510	
		LOWER LIMB		
75 t35		**Leg Length Discrepancy**	528 t 17-4	
76 t36		**Gait Derangement**	529 t 17-5	
77 t37		**Muscle Atrophy**	530 t 17-6	
77 t39		**Muscle Weakness**	532 t 17-8	
		Motion Impairment		
78 t40		**Hip**	537 t 17-9	
78 t41		**Knee**	537 t 17-10	
78 t42		**Ankle**	537 t 17-11	
78 t43		**Hindfoot**	537 t 17-12	
78 t44		**Hindfoot deformity**	537 t 17-13	
82 t61		**Toe Impairments**	537 t 17-14	
79-81 t48-59		**Ankylosis**	538-543 t 17-15 – t 17-30	
83 t62		**Arthritis(x-ray) + CMP**	544 t 17-31	
83 t63		**Amputations**	545 t 17-32	
85 t64		**Diagnostic Based Estimates**	546 t 17-33	
87 t65		**Hip Replacement (rating)**	548 t 17-34	
88 t66		**Knee Replacement (rating)**	549 t 17-35	
89 t68		**Skin Loss**	550 t 17-13	
		Nerve Deficits	552 t 17-37	
			482 t16-10(s)	484 t 16-11(m)
		SPINE		
110 t72		**L/S: DRE: Lumbar**	384 t 15-3	
110 t73		**C/Th: DRE Thoracic**	389 t 15-4	
111 t74		**Th/L: DRE Cervical**	392 t 15-5	
131 3 4		**Pelvis**	428 t 15-19	
			WCG 3rd Ed, page 33, table 4.3	

Table 16-1 Conversion of Impairment of the Digits to Impairment of the Hand*

% Impairment of Thumb	Hand	% Impairment of Index or Middle Finger	Hand	% Impairment of Ring or Little Finger	Hand
0 - 1	0	0 - 2	0	0 - 4	0
2 - 3	1	3 - 7	1	5 - 14	1
4 - 6	2	8 - 12	2	15 - 24	2
7 - 8	3	13 - 17	3	25 - 34	3
9 - 11	4	18 - 22	4	35 - 44	4
12 - 13	5	23 - 27	5	45 - 54	5
14 - 16	6	28 - 32	6	55 - 64	6
17 - 18	7	33 - 37	7	65 - 74	7
19 - 21	8	38 - 42	8	75 - 84	8
22 - 23	9	43 - 47	9	85 - 94	9
24 - 26	10	48 - 52	10	95 - 100	10
27 - 28	11	53 - 57	11		
29 - 31	12	58 - 62	12		
32 - 33	13	63 - 67	13		
34 - 36	14	68 - 72	14		
37 - 38	15	73 - 77	15		
39 - 41	16	78 - 82	16		
42 - 43	17	83 - 87	17		
44 - 46	18	88 - 92	18		
47 - 48	19	93 - 97	19		
49 - 51	20	98 - 100	20		
52 - 53	21				
54 - 56	22				
57 - 58	23				
59 - 61	24				
62 - 63	25				
64 - 66	26				
67 - 68	27				
69 - 71	28				
72 - 73	29				
74 - 76	30				
77 - 78	31				
79 - 81	32				
82 - 83	33				
84 - 86	34				
87 - 88	35				
89 - 91	36				
92 - 93	37				
94 - 96	38				
97 - 98	39				
99 - 100	40				

Table 16-2 Conversion of Impairment of the Hand to Impairment of the Upper Extremity*

Hand	Upper Extremity	Hand	Upper Extremity	Hand	Upper Extremity	Hand	Upper Extremity	Hand	Upper Extremity	Hand	Upper Extremity
0	0	18	16	36	32	54	49	72	65	90	81
1	1	19	17	37	33	55	50	73	66	91	82
2	2	20	18	38	34	56	50	74	67	92	83
3	3	21	19	39	35	57	51	75	68	93	84
4	4	22	20	40	36	58	52	76	68	94	85
5	5	23	21	41	37	59	53	77	69	95	86
6	5	24	22	42	38	60	54	78	70	96	86
7	6	25	23	43	39	61	55	79	71	97	87
8	7	26	23	44	40	62	56	80	72	98	88
9	8	27	24	45	41	63	57	81	73	99	89
10	9	28	25	46	41	64	58	82	74	100	90
11	10	29	26	47	42	65	59	83	75		
12	11	30	27	48	43	66	59	84	76		
13	12	31	28	49	44	67	60	85	77		
14	13	32	29	50	45	68	61	86	77		
15	14	33	30	51	46	69	62	87	78		
16	14	34	31	52	47	70	63	88	79		
17	15	35	32	53	48	71	64	89	80		

Upper Extremity	Whole Person	Upper Extremity	Whole Person	Upper Extremity	Whole Person	Upper Extremity	Whole Person	Upper Extremity	Whole Person
0	0	20	12	40	24	60	36	80	48
1	1	21	13	41	25	61	37	81	49
2	1	22	13	42	25	62	37	82	49
3	2	23	14	43	26	63	38	83	50
4	2	24	14	44	26	64	38	84	50
5	3	25	15	45	27	65	39	85	51
6	4	26	16	46	28	66	40	86	52
7	4	27	16	47	28	67	40	87	52
8	5	28	17	48	29	68	41	88	53
9	5	29	17	49	29	69	41	89	53
10	6	30	18	50	30	70	42	90	54
11	7	31	19	51	31	71	43	91	55
12	7	32	19	52	31	72	43	92	55
13	8	33	20	53	32	73	44	93	56
14	8	34	20	54	32	74	44	94	56
15	9	35	21	55	33	75	45	95	57
16	10	36	22	56	34	76	46	96	58
17	10	37	22	57	34	77	46	97	58
18	11	38	23	58	35	78	47	98	59
19	11	39	23	59	35	79	47	99	59
								100	60

*AMA Guides to the Evaluation of Permanent Impairment, 6th Edition

1	2
2	3	4
3	4	5	6
4	5	6	7	8
5	6	7	8	9	10
6	7	8	9	10	11	12
7	8	9	10	11	12	13	14
8	9	10	11	12	13	14	14	15
9	10	11	12	13	14	14	15	16	17
10	11	12	13	14	15	15	16	17	18	19
11	12	13	14	15	15	16	17	18	19	20	21
12	13	14	15	16	16	17	18	19	20	21	22	23
13	14	15	16	16	17	18	19	20	21	22	23	23	24
14	15	16	17	17	18	19	20	21	22	23	23	24	25	26
15	16	17	18	18	19	20	21	22	23	24	24	25	26	27	28
16	17	18	19	19	20	21	22	23	24	24	25	26	27	28	29	29
17	18	19	19	20	21	22	23	24	24	25	26	27	28	29	29	30	31
18	19	20	20	21	22	23	24	25	25	26	27	28	29	29	30	31	32	33
19	20	21	21	22	23	24	25	25	26	27	28	29	30	30	31	32	33	34	34
20	21	22	22	23	24	25	26	26	27	28	29	30	30	31	32	33	34	34	35	36
21	22	23	23	24	25	26	27	27	28	29	30	30	31	32	33	34	34	35	36	37	38
22	23	24	24	25	26	27	27	28	29	30	31	31	32	33	34	34	35	36	37	38	38	39
23	24	25	25	26	27	28	28	29	30	31	31	32	33	34	35	35	36	37	38	38	39	40	41
24	25	26	26	27	28	29	29	30	31	32	32	33	34	35	35	36	37	38	38	39	40	41	41	42
25	26	27	27	28	29	30	30	31	32	33	33	34	35	36	36	37	38	39	39	40	41	42	42	43	44
26	27	27	28	29	30	30	31	32	33	33	34	35	36	36	37	38	39	39	40	41	42	42	43	44	45	45
27	28	28	29	30	31	31	32	33	34	34	35	36	36	37	38	39	39	40	41	42	42	43	44	45	45	46	47
28	29	29	30	31	32	32	33	34	34	35	36	37	37	38	39	40	40	41	42	42	43	44	45	45	46	47	47	48
29	30	30	31	32	33	33	34	35	35	36	37	38	38	39	40	40	41	42	42	43	44	45	45	46	47	47	48	49	50
30	31	31	32	33	34	34	35	36	36	37	38	38	39	40	41	41	42	43	43	44	45	45	46	47	48	48	49	50	50	51
31	32	32	33	34	34	35	36	37	37	38	39	39	40	41	41	42	43	43	44	45	45	46	47	48	48	49	50	50	51	52	52
32	33	33	34	35	35	36	37	37	38	39	39	40	41	42	42	43	44	44	45	46	46	47	48	48	49	50	50	51	52	52	53	54
33	34	34	35	36	36	37	38	38	39	40	40	41	42	42	43	44	44	45	46	46	47	48	48	49	50	50	51	52	52	53	54	54	55
34	35	35	36	37	37	38	39	39	40	41	41	42	43	43	44	45	45	46	47	47	48	49	49	50	51	51	52	52	53	54	54	55	56	56
35	36	36	37	38	38	39	40	40	41	42	42	43	43	44	45	45	46	47	47	48	49	49	50	51	51	52	53	53	54	55	55	56	56	57	58
36	37	37	38	39	39	40	40	41	42	42	43	44	44	45	46	46	47	48	48	49	49	50	51	51	52	53	53	54	55	55	56	56	57	58	58	59
37	38	38	39	40	40	41	41	42	43	43	44	45	45	46	46	47	48	48	49	50	50	51	51	52	53	53	54	55	55	56	57	57	58	58	59	60	60
38	39	39	40	40	41	42	42	43	44	44	45	45	46	47	47	48	49	49	50	50	51	52	52	53	54	54	55	55	56	57	57	58	58	59	60	60	61	62
39	40	40	41	41	42	43	43	44	44	45	46	46	47	48	48	49	49	50	51	51	52	52	53	54	54	55	55	56	57	57	58	59	59	60	60	61	62	62	63
40	41	41	42	42	43	44	44	45	45	46	47	47	48	48	49	50	50	51	51	52	53	53	54	54	55	56	56	57	57	58	59	59	60	60	61	62	62	63	63	64
41	42	42	43	43	44	45	45	46	46	47	47	48	48	49	50	50	51	52	52	53	53	54	55	55	56	56	57	58	58	59	59	60	60	61	62	62	63	63	64	65	65
42	43	43	44	44	45	45	46	47	47	48	48	49	50	50	51	51	52	52	53	54	54	55	55	56	57	57	58	58	59	59	60	61	61	62	62	63	63	64	65	65	66	66
43	44	44	45	45	46	46	47	48	48	49	49	50	50	51	52	52	53	53	54	54	55	56	56	57	57	58	58	59	60	60	61	61	62	62	63	64	64	65	65	66	66	67	68
44	45	45	46	46	47	47	48	48	49	50	50	51	51	52	52	53	54	54	55	55	56	56	57	57	58	59	59	60	60	61	61	62	62	63	64	64	65	65	66	66	67	68	68	69
45	46	46	47	47	48	48	49	49	50	51	51	52	52	53	53	54	54	55	55	56	57	57	58	58	59	59	60	60	61	62	62	63	63	64	64	65	65	66	66	67	68	68	69	69	70
46	47	47	48	48	49	49	50	50	51	51	52	52	53	54	54	55	55	56	56	57	57	58	58	59	60	60	61	61	62	62	63	63	64	64	65	65	66	67	67	68	68	69	69	70	70	71
47	48	48	49	49	50	50	51	51	52	52	53	53	54	54	55	55	56	57	57	58	58	59	59	60	60	61	61	62	62	63	63	64	64	65	66	66	67	67	68	68	69	69	70	70	71	71	72
48	49	49	50	50	51	51	52	52	53	53	54	54	55	55	56	56	57	57	58	58	59	59	60	60	61	62	62	63	63	64	64	65	65	66	66	67	67	68	68	69	69	70	70	71	71	72	72	73
49	50	50	51	51	52	52	53	53	54	54	55	55	56	56	57	57	58	58	59	59	60	60	61	61	62	62	63	63	64	64	65	65	66	66	67	67	68	68	69	69	70	70	71	71	72	72	73	73	74
50	51	51	52	52	53	53	54	54	55	55	56	56	57	57	58	58	59	59	60	60	61	61	62	62	63	63	64	64	65	65	66	66	67	67	68	68	69	69	70	70	71	71	72	72	73	73	74	74	75	75
	1	**2**	**3**	**4**	**5**	**6**	**7**	**8**	**9**	**10**	**11**	**12**	**13**	**14**	**15**	**16**	**17**	**18**	**19**	**20**	**21**	**22**	**23**	**24**	**25**	**26**	**27**	**28**	**29**	**30**	**31**	**32**	**33**	**34**	**35**	**36**	**37**	**38**	**39**	**40**	**41**	**42**	**43**	**44**	**45**	**46**	**47**	**48**	**49**	**50**

The values are derived from the formula A + B(1 - A) = combined value of A and B, where A and B are the decimal equivalents of the impairment ratings. In the chart all values are expressed as percents. To combine any two impairment values, locate the larger of the values on the side of the chart and read along that row until you come to the column indicated by the smaller value at the bottom of the chart. At the intersection of the row and the column is the combined value.

For example, to combine 35% and 20%, read down the side of the chart until you come to the larger value, 35%. Then read across the 35% row until you come to the column indicated by 20% at the bottom of the chart. At the intersection of the row and column is the number 48. Therefore, 35% combined with 20% is 48%. Because of the construction of this chart, the larger impairment value must be identified at the side of the chart.

If three or more impairment values are to be combined, select any two and find their combined value as above. Then use that value and the third value to locate the combined value of all. This process can be repeated indefinitely, the final value in each instance being the combination of all the previous values. In each step of this process the larger impairment value must be identified at the side of the chart.

Note: If impairments from two or more organ systems are to be combined to express a whole person impairment, each must first be expressed as a whole person impairment percent.

	1	2	3	4	5	6	7	8	9	10	11	12	13	14	15	16	17	18	19	20	21	22	23	24	25	26	27	28	29	30	31	32	33	34	35	36	37	38	39	40	41	42	43	44	45	46	47	48	49	50
51	51	52	52	53	53	54	54	55	55	56	56	57	57	58	58	59	59	60	60	61	61	62	62	63	63	64	64	65	65	66	66	67	67	68	68	69	69	70	70	71	71	72	72	73	73	74	74	75	75	76
52	52	53	53	54	54	55	55	56	56	57	57	58	58	59	59	60	60	61	61	62	62	63	63	64	64	64	65	65	66	66	67	67	68	68	69	69	70	70	71	71	72	72	73	73	74	74	75	75	76	76
53	53	54	54	55	55	56	56	57	57	58	58	59	59	60	60	61	61	61	62	62	63	63	64	64	65	65	66	66	67	67	68	68	69	69	69	70	70	71	71	72	72	73	73	74	74	75	75	76	76	77
54	54	55	55	56	56	57	57	58	58	59	59	59	60	60	61	61	62	62	63	63	64	64	65	65	66	66	66	67	67	68	68	69	69	70	70	71	71	71	72	72	73	73	74	74	75	75	76	76	77	77
55	55	56	56	57	57	58	58	59	59	60	60	60	61	61	62	62	63	63	64	64	64	65	65	66	66	67	67	68	68	69	69	69	70	70	71	71	72	72	73	73	73	74	74	75	75	76	76	77	77	78
56	56	57	57	58	58	59	59	60	60	60	61	61	62	62	63	63	63	64	64	65	65	66	66	67	67	67	68	68	69	69	70	70	71	71	71	72	72	73	73	74	74	74	75	75	76	76	77	77	78	78
57	57	58	58	59	59	60	60	60	61	61	62	62	63	63	63	64	64	65	65	66	66	66	67	67	68	68	69	69	69	70	70	71	71	72	72	72	73	73	74	74	75	75	75	76	76	77	77	78	78	79
58	58	59	59	60	60	61	61	61	62	62	63	63	63	64	64	65	65	66	66	66	67	67	68	68	68	69	69	70	70	71	71	71	72	72	73	73	74	74	74	75	75	76	76	76	77	77	78	78	79	79
59	59	60	60	61	61	61	62	62	63	63	64	64	64	65	65	66	66	66	67	67	68	68	68	69	69	70	70	70	71	71	72	72	73	73	73	74	74	75	75	75	76	76	77	77	77	78	78	79	79	80
60	60	61	61	62	62	62	63	63	64	64	64	65	65	66	66	66	67	67	68	68	68	69	69	70	70	70	71	71	72	72	72	73	73	74	74	74	75	75	76	76	76	77	77	78	78	78	79	79	80	80
61	61	62	62	63	63	63	64	64	65	65	65	66	66	66	67	67	68	68	68	69	69	70	70	70	71	71	72	72	72	73	73	73	74	74	75	75	75	76	76	77	77	77	78	78	79	79	79	80	80	81
62	62	63	63	64	64	64	65	65	65	66	66	67	67	67	68	68	68	69	69	70	70	70	71	71	72	72	72	73	73	73	74	74	75	75	75	76	76	76	77	77	78	78	78	79	79	79	80	80	81	81
63	63	64	64	64	65	65	66	66	66	67	67	67	68	68	69	69	69	70	70	70	71	71	72	72	72	73	73	73	74	74	74	75	75	76	76	76	77	77	77	78	78	79	79	79	80	80	80	81	81	82
64	64	65	65	65	66	66	67	67	67	68	68	68	69	69	69	70	70	70	71	71	72	72	72	73	73	73	74	74	74	75	75	76	76	76	77	77	77	78	78	78	79	79	79	80	80	81	81	81	82	82
65	65	66	66	66	67	67	67	68	68	69	69	69	70	70	70	71	71	71	72	72	72	73	73	73	74	74	74	75	75	76	76	76	77	77	77	78	78	78	79	79	79	80	80	80	81	81	81	82	82	83
66	66	67	67	67	68	68	68	69	69	69	70	70	70	71	71	71	72	72	72	73	73	73	74	74	75	75	75	76	76	76	77	77	77	78	78	78	79	79	79	80	80	80	81	81	81	82	82	82	83	83
67	67	68	68	68	69	69	69	70	70	70	71	71	71	72	72	72	73	73	73	74	74	74	75	75	75	76	76	76	77	77	77	78	78	78	79	79	79	80	80	80	81	81	81	82	82	82	83	83	83	84
68	68	69	69	69	70	70	70	71	71	71	72	72	72	72	73	73	73	74	74	74	75	75	75	76	76	76	77	77	77	78	78	78	79	79	79	80	80	80	80	81	81	81	82	82	82	83	83	83	84	84
69	69	70	70	70	71	71	71	71	72	72	72	73	73	73	74	74	74	75	75	75	76	76	76	76	77	77	77	78	78	78	79	79	79	80	80	80	80	81	81	81	82	82	82	83	83	83	84	84	84	85
70	70	71	71	71	72	72	72	72	73	73	73	74	74	74	75	75	75	75	76	76	76	77	77	77	78	78	78	78	79	79	79	80	80	80	81	81	81	81	82	82	82	83	83	83	84	84	84	84	85	85
71	71	72	72	72	72	73	73	73	74	74	74	74	75	75	75	76	76	76	77	77	77	77	78	78	78	79	79	79	79	80	80	80	81	81	81	81	82	82	82	83	83	83	83	84	84	84	85	85	85	86
72	72	73	73	73	73	74	74	74	75	75	75	75	76	76	76	76	77	77	77	78	78	78	78	79	79	79	80	80	80	80	81	81	81	82	82	82	82	83	83	83	83	84	84	84	85	85	85	85	86	86
73	73	74	74	74	74	75	75	75	75	76	76	76	77	77	77	77	78	78	78	78	79	79	79	79	80	80	80	81	81	81	81	82	82	82	82	83	83	83	84	84	84	84	85	85	85	85	86	86	86	87
74	74	75	75	75	75	76	76	76	76	77	77	77	77	78	78	78	78	79	79	79	79	80	80	80	81	81	81	81	82	82	82	82	83	83	83	83	84	84	84	84	85	85	85	85	86	86	86	86	87	87
75	75	76	76	76	76	77	77	77	77	78	78	78	78	79	79	79	79	80	80	80	80	81	81	81	81	82	82	82	82	83	83	83	83	84	84	84	84	85	85	85	85	86	86	86	86	87	87	87	87	88
76	76	76	77	77	77	77	78	78	78	78	79	79	79	79	80	80	80	80	81	81	81	81	82	82	82	82	82	83	83	83	83	84	84	84	84	85	85	85	85	86	86	86	86	87	87	87	87	88	88	88
77	77	77	78	78	78	78	79	79	79	79	80	80	80	80	80	81	81	81	81	82	82	82	82	83	83	83	83	83	84	84	84	84	85	85	85	85	86	86	86	86	86	87	87	87	87	88	88	88	88	89
78	78	78	79	79	79	79	80	80	80	80	80	81	81	81	81	82	82	82	82	82	83	83	83	83	84	84	84	84	84	85	85	85	85	85	86	86	86	86	87	87	87	87	87	88	88	88	88	89	89	89
79	79	79	80	80	80	80	80	81	81	81	81	82	82	82	82	82	83	83	83	83	83	84	84	84	84	84	85	85	85	85	86	86	86	86	86	87	87	87	87	87	88	88	88	88	88	89	89	89	89	90
80	80	80	81	81	81	81	81	82	82	82	82	82	83	83	83	83	83	84	84	84	84	84	85	85	85	85	85	86	86	86	86	86	87	87	87	87	87	88	88	88	88	88	89	89	89	89	89	90	90	90
81	81	81	82	82	82	82	82	83	83	83	83	83	83	84	84	84	84	84	85	85	85	85	85	86	86	86	86	86	87	87	87	87	87	87	88	88	88	88	88	89	89	89	89	89	90	90	90	90	90	91
82	82	82	83	83	83	83	83	83	84	84	84	84	84	85	85	85	85	85	85	86	86	86	86	86	87	87	87	87	87	87	88	88	88	88	88	88	89	89	89	89	89	90	90	90	90	90	90	91	91	91
83	83	83	84	84	84	84	84	84	85	85	85	85	85	85	86	86	86	86	86	86	87	87	87	87	87	87	88	88	88	88	88	88	89	89	89	89	89	89	90	90	90	90	90	90	91	91	91	91	91	92
84	84	84	84	85	85	85	85	85	85	86	86	86	86	86	86	87	87	87	87	87	87	88	88	88	88	88	88	88	89	89	89	89	89	89	90	90	90	90	90	90	91	91	91	91	91	91	92	92	92	92
85	85	85	85	86	86	86	86	86	86	87	87	87	87	87	87	87	88	88	88	88	88	88	88	89	89	89	89	89	89	90	90	90	90	90	90	90	91	91	91	91	91	91	91	92	92	92	92	92	92	93
86	86	86	86	87	87	87	87	87	87	87	88	88	88	88	88	88	88	89	89	89	89	89	89	89	90	90	90	90	90	90	90	90	91	91	91	91	91	91	91	92	92	92	92	92	92	92	93	93	93	93
87	87	87	87	88	88	88	88	88	88	88	88	89	89	89	89	89	89	89	89	90	90	90	90	90	90	90	91	91	91	91	91	91	91	91	92	92	92	92	92	92	92	92	93	93	93	93	93	93	93	94
88	88	88	88	88	89	89	89	89	89	89	89	89	90	90	90	90	90	90	90	90	91	91	91	91	91	91	91	91	91	92	92	92	92	92	92	92	92	93	93	93	93	93	93	93	93	94	94	94	94	94
89	89	89	89	89	90	90	90	90	90	90	90	90	90	91	91	91	91	91	91	91	91	91	92	92	92	92	92	92	92	92	92	93	93	93	93	93	93	93	93	93	94	94	94	94	94	94	94	94	94	95
90	90	90	90	90	91	91	91	91	91	91	91	91	91	91	92	92	92	92	92	92	92	92	92	92	93	93	93	93	93	93	93	93	93	93	94	94	94	94	94	94	94	94	94	94	95	95	95	95	95	95
91	91	91	91	91	91	92	92	92	92	92	92	92	92	92	92	92	93	93	93	93	93	93	93	93	93	93	93	94	94	94	94	94	94	94	94	94	94	94	95	95	95	95	95	95	95	95	95	95	95	96
92	92	92	92	92	92	92	93	93	93	93	93	93	93	93	93	93	93	93	94	94	94	94	94	94	94	94	94	94	94	94	94	95	95	95	95	95	95	95	95	95	95	95	96	96	96	96	96	96	96	96
93	93	93	93	93	93	93	93	94	94	94	94	94	94	94	94	94	94	94	94	94	94	95	95	95	95	95	95	95	95	95	95	95	95	95	95	96	96	96	96	96	96	96	96	96	96	96	96	96	96	97
94	94	94	94	94	94	94	94	94	95	95	95	95	95	95	95	95	95	95	95	95	95	95	95	95	96	96	96	96	96	96	96	96	96	96	96	96	96	96	96	96	96	97	97	97	97	97	97	97	97	97
95	95	95	95	95	95	95	95	95	95	96	96	96	96	96	96	96	96	96	96	96	96	96	96	96	96	96	96	96	96	96	97	97	97	96	97	97	97	97	97	97	97	97	97	97	97	97	97	97	97	98
96	96	96	96	96	96	96	96	96	96	96	96	96	97	97	97	97	97	97	97	97	97	97	97	97	97	97	97	97	97	97	97	97	97	97	97	97	97	98	98	98	98	98	98	98	98	98	98	98	98	98
97	97	97	97	97	97	97	97	97	97	97	97	97	97	97	97	97	98	98	98	98	98	98	98	98	98	98	98	98	98	98	98	98	98	98	98	98	98	98	98	98	98	98	98	98	98	98	98	98	98	99
98	98	98	98	98	98	98	98	98	98	98	98	98	98	98	98	98	98	98	98	98	98	98	98	98	99	99	99	99	99	99	99	99	99	99	99	99	99	99	99	99	99	99	99	99	99	99	99	99	99	99
99	99	99	99	99	99	99	99	99	99	99	99	99	99	99	99	99	99	99	99	99	99	99	99	99	99	99	99	99	99	99	99	99	99	99	99	99	99	99	99	99	99	99	99	99	99	99	99	99	99	100

References

A number of textbooks and journal articles have been used as reference to produce this book, the two main books being:

1. Sinnatamby C. Last's anatomy, regional and applied. 10th ed. Edinburgh: Churchill Livingstone; 1999. ISBN 0 443 05611 0.
2. Solomon L, Warwick D, Nayagam S, Graham Apley A. Apley's system of orthopaedics and fractures. 9th ed. London: Hodder Arnold; 2010. ISBN: 9780340942086.

R. Pillemer, *Physical Signs in Orthopedic and Neurologic Disorders*, https://doi.org/10.1007/978-3-031-99529-3

Index

R. Pillemer, *Physical Signs in Orthopedic and Neurologic Disorders*,
https://doi.org/10.1007/978-3-031-99529-3

MIX
Papier aus verantwortungsvollen Quellen
Paper from responsible sources
FSC® C105338

If you have any concerns about our products,
you can contact us on
ProductSafety@springernature.com

In case Publisher is established outside the EU,
the EU authorized representative is:
Springer Nature Customer Service Center GmbH
Europaplatz 3, 69115 Heidelberg, Germany

Printed by Libri Plureos GmbH
in Hamburg, Germany